Spirituality
and Palliative Care

Spirituality

and Palliative Care

Social and Pastoral Perspectives   Edited by Bruce Rumbold

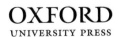

OXFORD
UNIVERSITY PRESS

OXFORD

UNIVERSITY PRESS

253 Normanby Road, South Melbourne, Victoria 3205, Australia

Oxford University Press is a department of the University of Oxford.
It furthers the University's objective of excellence in research, scholarship,
and education by publishing worldwide in

Oxford New York

Auckland Bangkok Buenos Aires Cape Town Chennai
Dar es Salaam Delhi Hong Kong Istanbul Karachi Kolkata
Kuala Lumpur Madrid Melbourne Mexico City Mumbai Nairobi
São Paulo Shanghai Singapore Taipei Tokyo Toronto

with an associated company in Berlin

OXFORD is a trade mark of Oxford University Press
in the UK and in certain other countries

National Library of Australia
Cataloguing-in-Publication data:

Spirituality and palliative care.

Includes index.
ISBN 0 19 551352 5.

1. Terminal care—Religious aspects. 2. Death—Religious aspects.
3. Death—Social aspects. I. Rumbold, Bruce D.

259.4175

Edited by Sandra Goldbloom Zurbo
Cover and text designed by Patrick Cannon
Indexed by Russell Brooks
Typeset by Kerry Cooke
Printed through Bookpac Production Services, Singapore

Contents

Acknowledgments

I would like to thank my friend and colleague, Allan Kellehear, who first suggested I develop the proposal for this book, then contributed to it, and encouraged me throughout the long period between contract and completion. Jill Henry as commissioning editor provided both unflagging support and constructive criticism, and I am most grateful to her and to all those at Oxford University Press who have been involved in its production.

The book marks for me a transition from teaching pastoral care in a theological school to my current role of teaching the sociology of death, dying, and palliative care in a university. Throughout the period of writing I worked half-time in each context, and the subtitle 'social and pastoral perspectives' reflects these dual involvements. I am grateful to my colleagues in the Theological School of Whitley College, Melbourne, for their friendship and support over a long period, and to Whitley College for providing study leave during which two chapters were written. I have enjoyed working with new colleagues in the School of Public Health, La Trobe University, particularly my fellow members of the Palliative Care Unit, and I look forward to being able to develop further some of the ideas put forward in this collection in my ongoing work there.

I am grateful to the contributors to this collection, some of them colleagues and friends of long standing, others relatively new acquaintances. All have been prompt in responding to the invitation to contribute and understanding of delays in completing the project. I am also grateful to my family, Jean and David, who not only bore patiently my preoccupations and weekend absences while I was finishing the task but also contributed respectively constructive comment and in-house entertainment.

Several chapters contain extracts from previously published works that should be acknowledged. Thanks are expressed to the *Guardian Weekly* for permission to include a quotation in chapter 2. Thanks are also expressed to Professor Ronald Anderson SJ of the Philosophy Department of Boston College for permission to quote material published on his web site.

Permission to use extracts from the third edition of Evan-Wentz' translation of *The Tibetan Book of the Dead* in chapter 9 has been granted by the publisher, Oxford University Press, New York. The extract from Elizabeth George's book *In Pursuit of the Proper Sinner* in chapter 10 is reproduced by permission of Hodder & Stoughton. The passage concerning Henri Nouwen in the same chapter is taken from *Wounded Prophet* by Michael Ford, published and copyright 1999 by Darton, Longman, & Todd, and used by permission of the publishers. Permission to use two brief quotations from *Caring: A Feminine Approach to Ethics and Moral Education,* by Nell Noddings, published by the University of California Press, 1984, has been given by the University of California Press.

Finally, I would like to thank Maggie May for permission to use the image on the cover of this book. Her drawing and collage is of detail from a medieval stone carving (1282–1310) in Valle Crucis Abbey, Llangollen, North Wales. This drawing, together with the drawing discussed in chapter 6, belongs to a series of art works made in Wales in 1993–99.

Bruce Rumbold
Melbourne, April 2002

Preface

Spirituality has a high profile today. Most bookshops have a section devoted to spirituality, in some cases incorporating traditional religious materials, in others separating religion from spirituality. Spirituality centres, sponsored by a variety of religious or healing traditions, are multiplying. Spirituality is an emerging theme in the professional and academic literatures of business, education, and healthcare, as well as in the curricula of training institutions. Spiritual needs find mention in government human service policies. Weekend newspapers and magazines advertise a bewildering diversity of therapies and programs for spiritual growth.

This book attempts to connect the social facts of this burgeoning interest in spirituality with contemporary discussions of spirituality in the healthcare field in general and palliative care in particular. It is a book about spirituality and palliative care, not merely spirituality in palliative care. It explores links between traditional religion and today's spirituality, reflects on traditional religious providers and contemporary spiritual carers and, in the light of this, develops some guidelines for spiritual practice in palliative care.

The aim of the collection is to contribute to a better-informed and more reflective debate about spirituality and spiritual care in palliative care practice. To date, most resources for the spiritual care of dying people either outline the personal and ritual requirements prescribed for the adherents of particular religious traditions or recommend strategies whereby a dying person can be supported to renew—or discover and affirm—his or her unique spiritual path. The former category tends to ignore the spirituality of those without formal religious belief or treats it as a secularised version of the dominant religion of their culture. The latter privatises spirituality, locating it in individual psychology and neglecting insights from religious traditions that speak to human spirituality in corporate or universal terms. Neither view gives sufficient attention to the social and cultural contexts in which palliative care—and contemporary approaches to spiritual care—are being practised. Nor do they give adequate recognition to the fact that the issues emerging in palliative care practice are frequently issues that relate to the whole of life, not merely the end of life; to debate them purely in the context of the last weeks or months of a person's lifetime can limit the resources and insights that should be brought to bear.

In seeking to complement and, hopefully, inform, such approaches, this collection includes contributions from theorists and practitioners representing various social and pastoral perspectives. There are no contributors from clinical practice disciplines in this collection, not because they have no contribution to make, but because this book is intended to complement the healthcare literature on the topic, currently dominated by clinical voices. The intention here is not to dismiss clinical perspectives but to point to a wider context, which must be taken into account in developing spiritual care.

There is no simple definition of spirituality common to these contributions. Lest this should seem to undermine the discussion, it should be noted from the outset that the same could be said of most contemporary discussions of, say, health. In fact, this very lack of consensus makes an important point. Definitions find general acceptance when an academic discipline or profession dominates that field. At this point, spirituality is a countervailing discourse, a way of talking, thinking, and acting that challenges the perspectives that have in the past been dominant: neither religion, nor, more recently, science, is able any longer to make authoritative pronouncements on the spiritual dimension.

Contributors here show both the discontinuities between spiritual care today and the religious care of previous eras, and ways in which religious understandings and processes can be resources for contemporary spirituality, even when that spirituality does not draw in any direct way upon religious texts, beliefs, rituals, or practices. Spirituality is seen as dealing with the same existential issues and fulfilling many of the same social functions that religion has done in past eras.

Some people acknowledge their spiritual nature but give it little further attention; others identify spirituality with a quest that is central to their lives. Some understand their spirituality through their connection with another who is perceived as a spiritual person—an advisor, a master, a director, or spiritual companion; others find spirituality inherent in a community and communal practices that take them beyond their own perceptions and concerns into a wider world of insight and experience.

❖

The chapters in this collection are arranged in three parts. Part 1, 'Exploring Spirituality', reviews a range of theoretical perspectives and resources that assist in understanding the contemporary scene. Part 2, 'Reflecting Upon Experience', contains first-person accounts ranging from people living with life-threatening illness and those involved in offering spiritual care to people with life-threatening illness. These latter accounts are dominated by the voices of pastoral care workers, not because they are the sole practitioners of spiritual care, but because they are the spiritual care practitioners whose voices are least in evidence in today's healthcare literature. The focus on experience in this part reflects a central contention of the book—that spiritual care becomes possible in mutual, human relationships. Part 3, 'Developing Responses', reintroduces social voices that discuss possibilities emerging in the field. The book concludes with Part 4, a brief section containing some guidelines that are, in effect, a position statement gleaned from this collection.

The book addresses issues involved in offering spiritual care in multicultural Western societies. It seeks to lay a foundation for the future in which the increasing religious and spiritual diversity that already characterises Western societies will appear in the palliative care practice of tomorrow.

Christianity is the major religious perspective represented within these contributions, not in an exclusive sense, but because palliative care is practised, for the most part, in countries where Christianity is the dominant religion and continues to permeate the society through public celebrations, holidays, and the stories and concepts associated with them.

This book does not discuss the specific contributions various religious traditions might make to the practice of spiritual care, or the spiritual needs of adherents of these traditions. Other literature is already available for this. Our interest here is in the nature and the dynamics of the spirituality brought to light in facing death and in caring for others facing death. Religious traditions are rich in resources for understanding and expressing this spirituality, but they are no longer the only frameworks through which contemporary spiritual experience is addressed.

Bruce Rumbold
Melbourne, 2002

Contributors

Paul Beirne has studied and worked in a number of countries, including for the last sixteen years, South Korea. He recently returned to Australia to take up the position of Dean and Director of Ministry Studies at the Melbourne College of Divinity.

Maryanne Confoy lectures in Religious Education and Practical Theology at the Jesuit Theological College and is President of the United Faculty of Theology in Melbourne, Victoria. She is Visiting Professor at the Institute of Religious Education and Pastoral Ministry at Boston College, USA. Among other published works, she is a contributing editor to *Freedom and Entrapment: Women Thinking Theology*, a collection of essays by leading Australian female theologians and academics, and *Morris West: A Writer and a Spirituality*. She is presently writing an authorised biography of Morris West. She has lectured and engaged in consultancy work in Australia, New Zealand, the USA, Ireland, the Pacific Islands, China, Bangladesh, India, and several South American countries.

Douglas Ezzy is a lecturer in the School of Sociology and Social Work at the University of Tasmania, Hobart, where he teaches qualitative methods and sociology of work. His research interests include unemployment and identity, HIV/AIDS, and New Age spirituality. He has published a number of articles in these areas, and recently co-authored, with Pranee Rice, *Qualitative Research Methods: A Health Focus*.

Jenny Hockey is senior lecturer in Health Studies in the School of Social Policy, University of Hull, UK. Her research interests are in the areas of ageing, terminal care, bereavement, and funeral management. Her books include *Experiences of Death, Growing Up and Growing Old: Ageing and Dependency in the Life Course*, and, with Elizabeth Hallam and Glennys Howarth, *Beyond the Body: Death and Social Identity*.

Bill Jenkins is the minister of Trinity Uniting Church in Perth, Western Australia. He has spent various periods over the past ten years in hospice ministry as chaplain and as consultant psychologist. He has a PhD in psychology and a Master's degree in theology, which was awarded for research into the experience of ministry to those who are dying. He is a member of the State Parole Board, an adjunct research fellow with the Faculty of Education, Curtin University of Technology, with interests in the education of children with special needs, and an associate of the John Curtin International Institute, with a focus on future studies in the psychosocial domain.

Allan Kellehear is foundation professor of palliative care and director of the Palliative Care Unit, Faculty of Health Sciences, La Trobe University, Melbourne, and an adjunct professorial fellow at the University of Melbourne Medical School. In 2000, he was British Academy visiting professor at the University of Bath and the Religious Experience Research Centre at Westminster College, Oxford. Among the fourteen books he has published, he is author of *Health Promoting Palliative Care* and *Eternity and Me*, and editor of *Death and Dying in Australia*.

Pamela McGrath is presently working as a University of Queensland senior research fellow, conducting a broad program of psychosocial research that is closely linked with a number of leading community organisations, including the Leukemia Foundation of Australia. In 1999, on the basis of international recognition of her work in psychosocial oncology and palliative care, she was named Eminent Scientist of the Year. Her research interests are in the area of the human experience of serious illness, with a particular focus on psycho-oncology, bioethics, spirituality, and palliative care. She has published over seventy articles in national and international journals and has written a number of books.

Maggie May is a printmaker, ceramicist, and sculptor, and has held part-time lecturing positions at RMIT University, the University of Melbourne, Lincoln Institute, and the Victorian College of the Arts. She has held four solo exhibitions and participated in more than thirty-five group exhibitions; she is represented in public and private collections in Australia, the United

Kingdom, Europe, and the USA and is the recipient of a number of awards. She has been a member of art committees and advisory groups. She is an artist in residence in the Yarra Valley for Parks Victoria.

Regina Millard is a member of the Religious Sisters of Charity, Australia. Following graduation from St Vincent's Hospital, Sydney, she worked for twenty years as a registered nurse, focusing on nurse education. After training at the Institute for Religious Formation, St Louis, Missouri, she began work in the palliative care field as a pastoral carer, first in 1993 with the Pastoral Care Team at Sacred Heart Hospice, Darlinghurst, Sydney, and then in Melbourne with Caritas Christi and Order of Malta Hospice Home Care Service, now part of Eastern Palliative Care. Her particular area of interest is pre- and post-bereavement care of adults and children within the family setting.

John E. Paver is a minister of the Uniting Church in Australia. Currently, he is professor of ministry at the Uniting Church Theological Hall, Parkville, Victoria, where he teaches theological field education and pastoral theology. For ten years he was head of the Pastoral Care Unit at the Peter MacCallum Cancer Institute and for three years chaplain to the Palliative Care Unit at the Heidelberg Repatriation Hospital, Heidelberg, Melbourne.

Bruce Rumbold is a senior lecturer in palliative care at La Trobe University. Before taking up this position he was professor of pastoral studies at Whitley College, whose theological school is affiliated with the Melbourne College of Divinity. He has postgraduate qualifications in solid-state physics, pastoral theology, and health sociology, and has published in all three fields. He is author of *Helplessness and Hope: Pastoral Care in Terminal Illness*.

Stan van Hooft is an associate professor of philosophy on the Burwood campus of Deakin University in Australia, with teaching experience in the School of Nursing. He is the author of *Caring: An Essay in the Philosophy of Ethics*, as well as numerous journal articles on moral philosophy, bioethics, and the nature of health and disease. He is also a co-author of *Facts and Values: An Introduction to Critical Thinking for Nurses*.

Part 1
Exploring Spirituality

Introduction

Most health sector attempts to assess spiritual need, to shape spiritual interventions, and to evaluate the effectiveness of those interventions follow one of four basic approaches. The first of these focuses on situations where people's ontological security is threatened or disintegrates as they experience radical changes arising from illness or injury. The second looks at the way people in changed circumstances, learning to live with chronic or life-threatening illness for example, review and revise their life stories to incorporate these changes and give meaning to their lives. The third is concerned with ways in which people may draw upon traditional religious resources to aid in their search for security or for meaning. The fourth considers how new spiritualities can support and inform quests that formerly may have been framed as religious concerns.

Part 1 provides a context for these approaches and shows how they complement each other. Chapter 1 looks at ways in which spiritual care has emerged as a focus within palliative care and how this interest in spirituality reflects that of Western society in general. The ambivalent relationship between this emergent spiritual interest and religious traditions is explored, underscoring a tension that persists within pastoral care practice itself, and between chaplains, pastoral care workers, and other professionals who also understand themselves to be providing spiritual care.

Maryanne Confoy (chapter 2) explores the historical continuity between traditional religious care and contemporary spiritual care by considering the pastoral tradition and the ways in which it has responded to the challenge of credible practice in a pluralistic world. Pastoral care is always practised in the face of the mystery of suffering and death: the palliative care context simply makes this explicit.

Stan van Hooft (chapter 3) presents an alternative perspective grounded in philosophical thought, arguing that spirituality may be located first and foremost in an encounter with the (human) other, and need not assume a belief in a transcendent realm or being. Relationship, not belief, is the place to start when exploring spirituality and spiritual care today.

The fourth and fifth chapters examine how spiritual resources are located within, and may be elicited from, people's experience. Jenny Hockey (chapter 4) describes how the resources to meet the threat of life-threatening illness may be found in a person's past, and how spiritual care is thus not something delivered by staff but a product of social interaction. Douglas Ezzy (chapter 5) outlines the narratives that people might develop through an encounter with life-threatening illness, in this case, HIV/AIDS, and shows how different narratives or patterns of meaning are constructed.

These chapters draw upon a wide range of resources and perspectives, but at least one clear theme unites them—spirituality is fundamentally relational.

1

From Religion to Spirituality

Bruce Rumbold

SPIRITUALITY AND HEALTHCARE

In Western societies before the 1970s, spiritual care was usually identified with religious care. This care was, for the most part, offered by practitioners authorised by particular religious groups or denominations. In hospitals religious care was optional, provided either by a hospital chaplain, a minister, a priest, or a rabbi from the local community. Those who did not actively participate in religious activities still expressed their spirituality by religious affiliation. That is, on admission to hospital, the vast majority of patients identified themselves with a religious denomination, indicating that belief was part of their social identity even if it was not expressed in consistent religious practice.

Denominational chaplains thus found themselves visiting and attempting to work with people whose nominal religious affiliation incorporated wide variations of belief and practice. With the increasing professionalism of chaplaincy, denominational appointments were superseded by ecumenical chaplaincies, while at the same time patients' religious affiliations became more diverse. The majority still acknowledged a religious connection, but it was often stated as Christian rather than denominational; at the same time, the number of those with no religious affiliation increased. Rather than limit themselves to a decreasing proportion of the inpatient population, chaplains began to look at ways of extending ministry to all. The rationale was that, while only some people were religious, spirituality was fundamental to humanity so that spiritual care was appropriate for all (Cobb & Robshaw 1998, p. ix). Chaplains, formed within and licensed by particular religious denominations, began to develop ways of operating beyond the boundaries not only of their denominations but also of their religious tradition.

At the same time renewed healthcare interest in spirituality was catalysed by the hospice movement that emerged in the 1970s. The earliest health literature on spiritual care came out of this movement, and it seems plausible to suggest that today's wider interest in spiritual care is associated in part with the mainstreaming of hospice care as palliative care. Contemporary palliative care is an outcome of the hospice movement, which emerged in the UK in the late 1960s and spread rapidly, largely in the English-speaking world, in the 1970s. Hospice reintroduced to Western society a public model for a good death, drawing upon both traditional resources in care for the dying—the tradition of hospitality in medieval religious communities—and modern medical techniques for symptom management (Clark 1998). Hospice was, in company with other communitarian ventures of the 1970s, a social experiment that was both radical and reforming (Abel 1986), radical in the sense that it returned to a premodern idea of care as exemplified in home-like environments, reforming in that it hoped to influence the way that care in general, not just care of the dying, was offered (Saunders et al. 1981). Its blending of traditional and modern resources blurred modernity's careful separation of public and private spheres (Walter 1994), producing an approach to care in which caring for patients also meant caring about them.

Seeking resources for a social understanding of a good death inevitably introduced religious agendas. Modern Western society had elected not to talk publicly about death, and consequently the resources available for renewed public discussion were religious for, in the West at least, death and eternal destiny were at the core of traditional religious concern. Thus the caring teams established to offer hospice care included as a matter of course ministers of religion. Indeed, religious groups were often in the forefront of promoting hospices in local communities, and healthcare personnel with active religious beliefs were strongly represented in hospice teams as a result of the movement's openness to spiritual concerns.

Hospice, however, quickly developed its preferred way of offering religious resources to its clients. Religious belief was not to be assumed or imposed, but the sorts of issues that might broadly be understood as religious concerns—core values, beliefs, attachments, directions—would be raised as opportunity allowed, and clients would be encouraged and supported to pursue them. Thus, Saunders, reflecting on the movement, places spirituality at the core when she says that 'Hospice has therefore adopted these principles—openness, mind together with heart, and a deep concern for the freedom of each individual to make his or her own journey towards their ultimate goals' (Saunders 1996, p. 319).

In the 1980s the hospice movement began to engage the mainstream healthcare services, a move that involved performance evaluation and a reframing of existing hospice programs as palliative care services. These services maintained much of the language and processes of the hospice movement, but the clinical systems with which they became increasingly enmeshed shaped priorities and directed procedures. Spiritual care, in an effort to conform or to be more accountable to the increasingly clinical interests and bureaucratic control of palliative care, developed standardised forms of spiritual assessment. Nevertheless, at a practice level, spirituality came to centre on the self. The content and the priorities of spiritual care were to be determined by the individual's experiences. A fundamental issue for spiritual care in palliative care, then, is whether clients on admission to the program bring with them an awareness of, and a capacity to articulate, their spirituality, or whether their admission to the program will be their first opportunity to become aware of, and perhaps begin to articulate, their spirituality. If the former, then presumably there will have been some movement to incorporate the reality of finitude and death; if the latter, eliciting an implicit spirituality may well precipitate further chaos if that spirituality turns out to be inadequate in the face of suffering and death.

As a consequence of these changing perceptions spiritual care has now moved beyond the bounds of religious institutions and chaplaincy departments. Within chaplaincy or pastoral care departments, more lay people are being appointed as formal religious accreditation is being replaced by professional and institutional accreditation. Further, increasing interest in spiritual care on the part of other healthcare disciplines is leaving religious practitioners at the margins (vandeCreek 1999). Spiritual care teams may include, in addition to or even in place of pastoral care workers, nurses, psychologists, occupational therapists, and social workers. We are now seeing a growing proportion of people (clients, patients, healthcare providers) who regard themselves as spiritual but not religious. No longer apparently passive nominal adherents of religious institutions, they take responsibility for their own spiritual understanding and practice. They may choose to consult with institutional spiritual care-givers, but they will not readily accede to being assessed, directed, or instructed by them.

There is a range of reasons for this revival of spirituality. Spiritual care provides a framework within which to acknowledge the religious needs that enter the secular health system through people from cultures that do not accept the separation of personal religion and the secular state. Spirituality restores the place of individuals and returns complexity to healthcare approaches that have in the past stereotyped or categorised people by their relationship with universalised norms, not according to their own experience. Spirituality can also be a tool for preserving or enhancing the status of a particular discipline or distinguishing it from another. Thus nursing rhetoric about holistic care obliges it to attend to spirituality. Occupational therapy uses spirituality as a representation of the individual uniqueness of each client. Politically, spirituality is increasingly correlated with ethical behaviour and, because of its flexibility, is a useful portmanteau term that caters for a range of people, from exponents of the New Age to those who are traditionally religious: unlike religion, spirituality lacks a clear, generally accepted definition (Hay & Nye 1998).

Spirituality is a means for challenging the authority of medical science and of regaining some agency, some autonomy, in situations that otherwise would be treated as scientifically determined. It may well be that language about spirituality has had to be revived because even the ostensibly person-centred disciplines of psychology and psychiatry have withdrawn into more scientific, less person-centred, frames. That is, spirituality appears as the shadow side of clinical science and provides a bridge between mainstream clinical disciplines and the complementary therapies that are increasing in social acceptability.

Thus current healthcare discussions bear the marks of their hospice origins and hospice's assimilation into palliative care. Hospice's appeal to traditional resources returns death and destiny to public discussion and its reform agenda continues to appear in the approaches that use spirituality as a means to challenge and critique clinical approaches to care. Palliative care's ambivalence about religion is reflected in the changing personnel involved in spiritual care. What we see as hospice transforms into palliative care and finds its place in the healthcare system, representing in microcosm the social transformation of religion in Western society today.

SPIRITUALITY AND WESTERN SOCIETY

Before the modern era religion was an integral aspect of culture, that is, people's culture determined their religious affiliation. It was only in the seventeenth century, as options emerged with the fragmentation of religious authority during the Renaissance and Reformation (Beyer 1998), that religion became differentiated from culture. As religious authority declined, that of science increased, ushering in the modern era in which scientific knowledge and method has been dominant. This dominance has been mediated through social institutions that have allied themselves with science, the healthcare system being one example of this. The authority given to science's empirical, quantifiable, and universal knowledge lessened the influence of other approaches to knowledge and relegated much of it to the realm of private preference. Thus at the height of the modern era public life was secular, and spirituality was identified as the private religious choice of individuals.

Renewed public interest in spirituality does not, however, come from a return to religious authority but from the increasing authority of the self. The general, objective, universal, rational ideals privileged by science are again being challenged by local, timely, subjective, personal experience (Toulmin 1990). It is not only in individual life but also in the life of communities and societies that qualities that have in the past been marginalised make their claim for attention, often at the expense of the forces that marginalised them in the first place. This happened to dominant religion when fledgling science mounted its challenge. It is happening now for science as individual experience challenges the normalising tendency of scientific approaches. Individual preferences, beliefs, and practices are now made public and are accepted in ways unthinkable at the height of the modern era. No longer need they be justified by reference to external—read scientific or religious—authority; self-assertion or personal testimony can be legitimation enough.

Spirituality has become one of the vehicles for asserting personal authority and identity in the face of scientific authority that neglected the subjective, relational, and transcendent aspects of identity. When, however, this spirituality draws upon religious forms it does so in ways that are different from the past. Today, diverse religious traditions are available to individuals in their search for meaning. Klass comments that 'our grandparents, for the most part, were born into one religion. Our children are born into a world in which all religions have a voice' (1999, p. 21). With this change has come a reversal of authority—from the authority of a specific tradition over individuals to that of the individual over religious traditions.

This reversal has been mediated by science. In traditional society, religion emphasised human insufficiency in order to provide religious answers (Kolakowski 1982). Modern society emphasised technological achievements made possible through scientific advancement, and technological success engendered a new optimism about human possibilities, albeit in a material sense. In the postmodern era we are beginning to see that, while scientific achievement has enabled us to manage some risks, shown particularly in increased longevity in the Western world, it has generated others—the global arms race and the cost of technology to the environment principal among them. Recognition of the insufficiency of science has not, however, led to a return to traditional religious pessimism concerning human possibilities (except in some millenarian cults, whose marginal nature shows them to be out of step with the times). Rather, modern optimism seems to have transformed itself into a faith in human potential to overcome or reach beyond the limitations of both religion and science. This optimism takes many different forms. Some see Western society as being on the threshold of a New Age which will be marked by self-determination and freedom. Some more modestly suggest that new forms of spirituality will need to arise if postmodernity is to contain the utter openness of modernity (Giddens 1990). Still others hope for new possibilities coming about through the transformation of old authorities: religion revived, or scientific understanding of human consciousness advancing to the point where we will be able to understand and, presumably, bring under control, those unruly aspects that have disrupted modernity (Crick 1994). This change of consciousness is shown not only in the rise of new spiritualities but also in the way previous authorities—religion and science—are regarded and have come to regard themselves.

The revival of spirituality clearly is linked with the appearance of the New Age movement, although this has been a symptom, rather than the source, of revival. In fact, to use the term 'movement' probably implies too great a coherence to the New Age. The organisations and ideas gathered under this banner are hugely diverse, and there is strenuous debate among both participants and spectators as to who actually belongs there. Nevertheless, broad characteristics of the movement are relatively clear (Heelas 1996). At the core of the New Age is what Heelas calls self-spirituality, expressed in three main ideas. First, life is not as it should be because we have been indoctrinated by mainstream society and culture. Second, new life—perfection—can only be found through paying attention to the essential spiritual self, to an inner spirituality that contrasts with the ego developed by the demands of society. Third, our inner potential is naturally realised once the great stumbling block of the ego has been dealt with (1996, pp. 18–20).

Diversity within the New Age movement comes about through differing emphases and methods of implementing these ideas. New Age groups run the full gamut of attitudes to mainstream society, from those who reject it as inevitably contaminating through to those who believe it can be developed in fresh ways. The goal of the former is to experience the best of inner spirituality, while that of the latter is to experience the best of the outer world. Thus at one end of the spectrum the pursuit of spirituality brings about detachment from the world, while at the other, spirituality becomes a tool for empowering people to achieve worldly success. As with most distributions, the majority can be found in the middle, between the purists and the empowerers (Heelas 1996, p. 32), seeking a harmony that will allow them to experience the best of both worlds. The New Age is variously an experience beyond society, a possibility that can be glimpsed within today's society, and a goal towards which society, once enlightened, can move.

A similar diversity is found in disciplines or practices by which people are invited to achieve and live out their changed consciousness. These range from physical methods for altering consciousness (fasting, drugs) to reflective disciplines (meditation, reading), practised either alone or in community. Where practice is communal, the context can range from the total environment of an enclosed residential community to a regular or occasional group meeting. It is here too that diverse resources come into play. There have been, and continue to be, strong religious influences within the New Age. The majority of these have been drawn from Eastern religions and traditional spiritualities (Native American in particular), Christian resources having been seen as fatally compromised by their contribution to and participation in mainstream Western capitalist society. More recently, however, there has been a revival of strands of spirituality similar to those from the East, such as Celtic spirituality and creation spirituality among Christians, Kabbalah, and related mystical traditions among Jews.

While some of the spiritualities that use religious resources ignore scientific world views, others endeavour to embrace them. Some of these postulate a convergence of religious and scientific worldviews through a common cosmology, usually illustrated by exploring conceptual similarities between quantum mechanical representations of matter and mystical beliefs concerning the nature of the universe (Capra 1983, for example). Others, such as Wilber's spectrum psychology (1977), extrapolate scientific systems to incorporate data and approaches previously regarded as mystical or religious. Yet other literature, less concerned with building grand narratives, discusses the convergence of mind and spirit in conversations between psychiatry and religion, or the implications of mind–body approaches for medicine. Further accounts are essentially autobiographical, outlining the authors' search for meaning when scientific or clinical formation and experience proved less than adequate in the face of major life issues (Cole 1999; Moore 1994).

Again, this is a diverse literature, but a common theme is connectedness. The categorisation and separations sought by modernity are challenged, and new connections are explored. One strong theme is ecological integrity, from which a revised understanding of transcendence begins to emerge. Many —although not all—traditional religious cosmologies see creation as transcended by the divine who (or which) stood beyond as well as within creation yet related in essentially personal ways with humans as the crown of that creation. In contrast, many contemporary cosmologies emphasise the way we humans are transcended by the ecosystems in which we participate. Our participation has a spiritual dimension—it provides meaning, a place, a purpose, a relationship with powers beyond ourselves—but this transcendence is not necessarily theistic. There is no need to postulate a deity transcending the ecosystem; to experience oneself as being transcended is not necessarily interpreted in religious terms.

New Age emphases can be incorporated within continuing institutional practice of religion, while New Age groups can engage institutional religions in a variety of ways. They may attempt to reach behind the religious experiences of one or many traditions to find a common unifying core. They may reject or replace a religious understanding and religious practice. Similarly, most scientific approaches are no longer merely dismissive of religious and spiritual perspectives. Although some assume that a material basis for spirituality will at length be demonstrated, others are open to the idea of a 'fifth dimension' (Hick 1999) that transcends physical reality.

FROM RELIGION TO SPIRITUALITY

The outline above is based upon trends in popular and professional literature, not the findings of social surveys. Nevertheless, today's interest in spirituality runs counter to the expectations of the large majority of 1960s and 1970s social theorists, who confidently predicted that secularism would increasingly characterise Western societies. Secularisation theory was developed from studies of the decline of institutional religion in Western, particularly European, societies. It has in many respects persuasively interpreted this decline and correctly predicted continuing reductions in participation in traditional religious institutions. The theory is, however, challenged by data from North America and developing nations in Asia, Africa, and South America, where social change may be associated with increased participation in religious activities. Religion does not inevitably decline as a society develops technologically. Nor does the decline of institutional religion in Europe and elsewhere imply the disappearance of belief or of spiritual practices, as indicated above. Survey data show a considerable proportion of people in a 'believing but not belonging' category (Davie 2000). Some interpret this gap as simply an artefact of the transition, asserting that in due course reported belief too will decline (Bruce 1995). Others argue that what secularisation theory interprets as the decline of religion is actually the deregulation of religion (Lyon 2000), that is, religious resources are becoming aspects of the culture, so that beliefs and practices associated with religious institutions are no longer under their control but may be adopted or adapted as individuals so choose. Religious, or spiritual, belief now appears to be a matter of personal choice. Unlike in traditional forms of social organisation, where religion was implicit in culture, or modern forms where a private choice could be made between particular forms of religious affiliation, individuals now may draw upon a range of religious and other resources to fashion a spirituality that fulfils functions that may previously have been discharged by religion.

This interpretation of course depends upon further assumptions that are also subject to debate, principally, whether as human beings we have *a priori* religious needs to be met, or whether in the future the needs currently met by religion, whether institutional or deregulated, will be met in other ways from other resources. Answers vary. Eliade (Hick 1999, p. 3) asserts that the sacred is an element in the structure of human consciousness, not a stage in the history of consciousness, and Rappaport (1999) sees religion to be fundamental in the making of humanity. In contrast to these anthropological assertions, Crick (1994) believes that eventually a fully scientific understanding of human consciousness will remove the need for religious interpretations of human nature and ethical behaviour, placing them instead on a thoroughly scientific footing.

Crick's framing of the issue as a choice between religion and science illustrates a fundamental problem facing any discussions of spirituality in the healthcare sector. While there is ample evidence of a new approach to spirituality in contemporary Western culture, healthcare discussions often continue to be framed, or assessed, in terms of the modernist debate between science and religion. In this debate the question is one of authority: which perspective can interpret the other? Postmodernists ask a different question: what use can I make of these different kinds of knowledge? The underlying issue shifts from commitment to the truth to self-development through consumption of knowledge and experience.

It is clear that postulating a spiritual nature for humankind continues to raise issues for a range of disciplines. Whether spirituality undergirds or precedes religion, or is constructed by it, has implications for biological, psychological, and social disciplines (Hay & Nye 1998). It is an issue also for traditional religious worldviews. Innate human religiousness leaves entirely open the crucial question of whether or not there is a transcendent reality to which religion is a response (Hick 1999, p. 3).

A FUTURE FOR (RELIGIOUS) BELIEF?

Do the spiritualities emerging today represent new directions for religious belief? Are they residual fragments of those beliefs that now are in the process of disappearing? Is a new age dawning, or is the hard-won scientific knowledge of the past now under threat? While we are not in any position to offer definitive answers to these questions, our willingness to consider them is important. Whether we see today's interest in spirituality as a last vestige of a superstitious past, the foreshadowing of a radically different future, or one aspect of a continuing human quest, will shape the way we engage with the new spiritualities. The questions invite us to look further at continuities and discontinuities between religion and spirituality.

James Thrower (1999) identifies three major religious theories of religion plus a further four naturalistic theories. The religious theories are:
- first, that religion is human response to the revealed word of God (a claim central to the Semitic religions—Judaism, Christianity, and Islam, for example)
- second, that religion is based in human experience of a transcendent reality (represented by the mystical tradition of many religions, both East and West)
- third, that religion arises from a philosophical understanding of the world—it makes and supports truth claims about reality.

Naturalistic theories focus on explanations alternative to these three: that religion is
- a human construct (presented by a range of philosophical critiques)
- a primitive error (an anthropological critique)

- a psychological construct (thus Feuerbach, Nieztsche, and Freud), or
- a social construct (Marx, Engels, Durkheim, and Weber).

At its starkest the contrast is between religious claims that religion offers access to basic knowledge concerning our human condition and naturalistic claims that religion masks or conceals such knowledge. This contrast between theories can, however, be overdrawn; in practice, to espouse one theory does not require rejecting all others out of hand. Religions of revelation also have a place for mystical experience and philosophical enquiry. Further, many believers recognise the validity of certain naturalistic critiques, for example, most pastoral care practitioners would recognise that religion may mask immaturity and illness, and thus support illusion, while maintaining that religion may also be a way to maturity and wholeness. Similarly, many who mount a naturalistic critique of religion do not see that critique as explaining away religious behaviour or denying a spiritual dimension to human existence. Religion may be culturally constructed, but that does not necessarily imply that it cannot express essential elements of human identity.

Continuity between religion and spirituality can at least be inferred from the fact that the new spiritualities face critique from the same constructionist or evolutionary theories that challenge religion. The secularist critics include both those principally concerned to eliminate any role for religion in public life and those who see the new spiritualities as representing continuing reluctance to embrace the self-reliance offered by science. For the former the individualism of the new spiritualities is more acceptable than the institutional forms of religion, and their opposition is less trenchant than that of the latter scientific rationalists. The persuasiveness of the rationalists' arguments, however, has waned. Dismissing religion or spirituality on the grounds that it is socially or culturally constructed loses force when it can equally be argued that the critiquing perspective is itself socially constructed. That is, pluralism replaces the dominant ideologies of the past, and neither science nor religion has the social authority to legitimate or dismiss the new spiritualities.

Continuity between new spiritualities and traditional religions is most evident in the way the new spiritualities continue to deal with what has been the core business of religion as it relates with individuals—providing meaning, developing practices that create and nurture transformative experiences, forming communities of practice. Not that any simple convergence, even of the differing strands of religious tradition, is in sight. As Ward remarks, 'the differences between religious traditions are nowhere clearer than in their views of human nature' and, 'since these views span the whole spectrum of possibilities, it would seem absurd to say that they all really agree' (1998, p. 324). Ward does, however, go on to identify features that are common to the diverse religious views he has explored.

> They all see the material world, as it is now constituted, as inherently unsatis-factory. They all propose some better, or truer, form of existence, which can be obtained through religious practice. And they all construe that practice in terms of a rather ascetic or disciplined attitude to the material world, and the cultivation of conscious states of bliss, wisdom and compassion. They all seek liberation from selfish greed, and experience of a selfless and blissful state or condition (1998, p. 324).

The same can be said of the majority of new spiritualities (Heelas 1996).

Ward points to the 'forced choices' imposed by the logical incompatibility of religious traditions on matters such as the self, suggesting that this makes it necessary to commit ourselves to a particular tradition of disclosure (1998, p. 326). But it may be that his analysis puts too high a value on rational coherence. In practice people seem to have little trouble in drawing upon ele-ments of several faith traditions, largely because practices have become divorced from the beliefs that formed them (Gilmour 2000; Groff 1999). Postmodern spirituality need not submit to the organising logic or rituals of religion or science. The (socially constructed) self is the new authority, giving dispensation from all requirements other than personal preference.

Discontinuity between religion and emerging spiritualities is most evident at the institutional level. Traditional religious institutions are, by and large, less than hospitable to new religious movements and individualistic forms of belief (see, for example, the range of Christian responses to the New Age in Ferguson 1993). Discontinuity is there also in the increasing authority of personal exper-ience over institutional legitimation. Some forms of religion will not admit the possibility of new insights that challenge received wisdom, while some new spir-itualities remain unashamedly scientific in their insistence that new knowledge must replace the old. Such positions tend to issue in mutual caricaturing: reli-gious people are portrayed as unable to think for themselves, while non-religiously spiritual people are labelled as self-indulgent or self-absorbed. In practice, critical thinkers can be found among religious adherents, and included among those who no longer practise religion are people who have left church, mosque, or synagogue in order to preserve or enhance their spiritual lives.

This shift of authority from religious institutions to the self has taken place both within and without organised religion. Wuthnow (1998) identifies a shift in American society from religious life as 'dwelling' within a particular religious tradition to 'seeking' among many possibilities. A consequence of this is that spiritual practice is less and less predictable on the basis of people's expressed beliefs or institutional participation. 'Spirituality comes to be seen as an aspect of the autonomous subject' (Lyon 2000, p. 51). Spirituality is expressed in the 'meaning-routes' that people follow from day to day, bringing together their ethnic and religious backgrounds in the context of the choices and constraints they face. Ammerman argues that it is now not a question of who is religious and how religious they might be, but 'how religious rhetorics and practices are enacted and how they are situated in various organisational contexts' (1997). We need, then, to focus on how people make a life rather than just on how they make sense (Lyon 2000, p. 52). Practice, more than formally articulated belief, becomes central to understanding spirituality.

It seems that any contrast between religion as composed of global institutions and new spiritualities as grassroots individual initiatives is overdrawn. Religious adherents are often much more flexible than institutional forms might suggest, while new spiritualities are more organised than might appear at first glance (Chryssides 1999). It is still a matter for debate as to whether the deregulated fragments of traditional beliefs will coalesce in new patterns to become new collective forms of belief. Hervieu-Léger (2000) for one suggests that this will indeed be the case, and that new communities are already emerging. Such collectives will be organised around common beliefs and practices, although whether they will bear any resemblance to the religious institutions of the past is another matter.

In summary, it appears that there is good reason to assume some continuity between religion and spirituality in both content and function. That is, spirituality continues to draw upon religious concepts and resources, and to address the same sorts of questions in people's lives. Discontinuity appears at the level of authority and practice. Belief for a majority of people in the Western world is no longer regulated through religious institutions, while even those who continue to participate in religious institutions resist such regulation. Further, the shift in spiritual practice from dwelling to seeking (Wuthnow 1998) reflects a shift in Western social identity from producer to consumer (Bauman 1998), raising the question whether Wuthnow's terminology is adequate. Seeking has overtones of a religious past, of the tradition of pilgrimage. But in a consumer society, seeking may look more like tourism than pilgrimage; the focus is on sampling a variety of spiritual experience rather than adopting particular spiritual pathways (Lyon 2000, p. 109).

Spiritualities that focus on consumption and self-direction may well struggle in the face of death. Death brings an end to consumption—at least to most forms of consumption—and challenges self-direction. Thus the spiritual practices that have supported people's lives may be unable to support them in their dying. Heelas expresses a similar concern: 'The more that people come to treat religion as a consumer item, the less likely they are to be attracted to the "real" thing. It might well be claimed that the omens for *religion*—as something requiring discipline, obedience, the exercise of the supra-individual, authorial—are not too good' (1998, p. 16).

Bauman, however, suggests that the postmodern investment in immediate experience is also capable of embracing death: 'Death, deployed once by religion as a kind of extraordinary event which nevertheless imparts meaning to all ordinary events, has turned itself into an ordinary event—even if, admittedly, the last in the chain of ordinary events, the last episode in the string of episodes' (1998, p. 66). He appears to be pointing to yet another reversal. Religious views have focused upon the presence of death in the midst of life as a means for living in the moment. Contemporary spiritualities focus on life in the midst of death, seeing dying as one more experience to be embraced.

SPIRITUAL CARE

Some of this discussion may seem to have taken us a long way from palliative care concerns about spiritual care. However, current practices in spiritual care both contribute to and reflect the social changes we have been reviewing here. If modernity marginalised death in reaction to the impossible demands of religious obsession with death (Delumeau 1990), then palliative care, bringing modernity back into dialogue with death, may yet make a significant contribution to an emerging postmodern spirituality.

Clearly, we live in transitional times such that today spirituality encompasses both religious beliefs and religious-like behaviours not associated with formal religious participation. Talking about spirituality thus continues to be problematic, as language shifts uneasily between religious and psychological terminology. The contentious part of the way 'spiritual' is being used in some places is its extension to incorporate worldviews that acknowledge the other, but not necessarily any transcendent reality, a point examined in detail in the following chapter. It is clear, however, that spirituality as a concept offers ways of looking at the world that resist the stereotyping inherent in much professional practice and can restore some sense of agency to the person. Variety is inherent in spirituality, and each individual may draw, in his or her own way, upon the various aspects of faith traditions or new religious ideas. This in itself is a challenge to healthcare systems that rely upon normalisation and standardised practices to offer care. Spiritual care refuses to be conformed to a standardised or fact-file approach, even for those who maintain a connection with formal religion.

An understanding of religious traditions and of the ways these traditions are being reinterpreted and accessed in contemporary society is vital. While each individual may express his or her spirituality in unique ways, the building blocks of belief and the modes in which belief is expressed are culturally shaped. The need for a theory-building approach is evident (Kellehear 2000) and this must take account of the continuity between religious belief and the contemporary spiritualities. Such continuity immediately raises questions about the separation between spirituality and religion assumed by much of the healthcare spirituality literature.

By ignoring the insights of religious studies, the healthcare literature's discussion of spirituality has all too often reflected the inadequacies of clinical ways of knowing. While the presenting reason for discussing spirituality is that care needs to be holistic, the discussions themselves often betray a clinical mindset. Far from exploring the range and complexity of human wholeness, they reflect individualism and problem-oriented reductionism. Spiritual need becomes closely aligned with emotional need, and the identified goals of spiritual care serve clinical interests. Thus an individual's spirituality is legitimate when it reinforces clinical goals, but suspect when it produces noncompliance and disrupts clinical process. The emphasis on each person's ability and responsibility to create his or her own meaning needs also to be challenged. This consumerist understanding—that it is now all a matter of personal preference—is inadequate insofar as it avoids scrutiny of the way personal perceptions and the choices available are shaped socially. Individual choices align us with communities of practice. Fundamentally, in far too much of the healthcare literature, scientific ways of knowing are substituted for the ways of knowing attested to in religious experience.

Changes in spiritual practices are also being reflected in the diversification and deregulation of pastoral care and spiritual care. How spiritual care should be carried out, and who should offer it, continue to be ongoing issues. For palliative care practice a particular question is whether end-of-life spiritual care can make up for rest-of-life neglect of spirituality. Currently, much end-of-life spiritual care seems to involve reorganising the fragments of earlier religiosity, an exercise that increases in difficulty the later after diagnosis these spiritual issues are confronted.

The inadequacies are reasonably easy to identify, solutions less easy to articulate. In the following chapters, we will attempt to move beyond problems to possibilities, which will involve us in shifting our focus beyond the clinic to the community.

REFERENCES

Abel, E. K. 1986, 'The hospice movement: Institutionizing innovation', *International Journal of Health Services*, vol. 16, pp. 71–85.

Ammerman, N. 1997, 'Religious choice and religious vitality' in L. Young, *Rational Choice Theory and Religion: Summary and Assessment*, Routledge, New York.

Bauman, Z. 1998, 'Postmodern religion', in P. Heelas, *Religion, Modernity and Postmodernity*, Blackwell, London, pp. 58–78.

Beyer, P. 1998, 'The city and beyond as dialogue: Negotiating religious authenticity in global society', *Social Compass*, vol. 45, pp. 67–79.

Bruce, S. 1995, *Religion in Modern Britain*, Oxford University Press, Oxford.

Capra, F. 1983, *The Turning Point: Science, Society and the Rising Culture*, Fontana, London.

Chryssides, G. 1999, *Exploring New Religions*, Cassell, London.

Clark, D. 1998, 'Originating a movement: Cicely Saunders and St Christopher's Hospice 1957–67', *Mortality*, vol. 3, pp. 43–63.

Cobb, M. & Robshaw, V. (eds) 1998, *The Spiritual Challenge of Health Care*, Churchill Livingstone, Edinburgh.

Cole, R. 1999, *Mission of Love: A Physician's Personal Journey Towards a Life Beyond*, Lothian Books, Melbourne.

Crick, F. 1994, *The Astonishing Hypothesis: The Scientific Search for the Soul*, Simon & Schuster, New York.

Davie, G. 2000, 'Religion in modern Britain: Changing sociological assumptions', *Sociology*, vol. 34, pp. 113–28.

Delumeau, J. 1990, *Sin and Fear: The Emergence of a Western Guilt Culture 13th–18th Centuries*, St Martin's Press, New York.

Ferguson, D. 1993, *New Age Spirituality: An Assessment*, Westminster John Knox Press, Louisville.

Giddens, A. 1990, *The Consequences of Modernity*, Stanford University Press, Stanford.

Gilmour, P. 2000, 'Spiritual borderlands: Practising more than a single religious tradition', *Listening: Journal of Religion and Culture*, vol. 35, no. 1, pp. 17–24.

Groff, L. 1999, 'Crossing boundaries: Spiritual journeys in search of the sacred', *Concilium*, no. 2, pp. 116–24.

Hay, D. & Nye, R. 1998, *The Spirit of the Child*, Fount, London.

Heelas, P. 1996, *The New Age Movement*, Blackwell, Oxford.

—— 1998, *Religion, Modernity and Postmodernity*, Blackwell, Oxford.

Hervieu-Léger, D. 2000, *Religion as a Chain of Memory*, Polity Press, Cambridge.

Hick, J. 1999, *The Fifth Dimension: An Exploration of the Spiritual Realm*, Oneworld Publications, Oxford.

Kellehear, A. 2000, 'Spirituality in palliative care: A model of needs', *Palliative Medicine*, vol. 14, pp. 149–55.

Klass, D. 1999, *The Spiritual Lives of Bereaved Parents*, Brunner/Mazel, Philadelphia.

Kolakowski, L. 1982, *Religion: If There is No God ... On God, the Devil, Sin and Other Worries of the So-called Philosophy of Religion*, Fontana, London.

Lyon, D. 2000, *Jesus in Disneyland: Religion in Postmodern Times*, Polity Press, Cambridge.

Moore, T. 1994, *Echoes of the Early Tides: A Healing Journey*, HarperCollins, Sydney.

Rappaport, R. 1999, *Ritual and Religion in the Making of Humanity*, Cambridge University Press, Cambridge.

Saunders, C. 1996, 'Hospice', *Mortality*, vol. 1, pp. 317–22.

——, Summers, D., & Teller, N. (eds) 1981, *Hospice: The Living Idea*, Edward Arnold, London.

Thrower, J. 1999, *Religion: The Classical Theories*, Georgetown University Press, Washington, DC.

Toulmin, S. 1990, *Cosmopolis: The Hidden Agenda of Modernity*, University of Chicago Press, Chicago.

vandeCreek, L. 1999, 'Professional chaplaincy: An absent profession?', *Journal of Pastoral Care*, vol. 53, pp. 417–32.

Walter, T. 1994, *The Revival of Death*, Routledge, London.

Ward, K. 1998, *Religion and Human Nature*, Clarendon Press, Oxford.

Wilber, K. 1977, *The Spectrum of Consciousness*, Theosophical Publishing House, Wheaton.

Wuthnow, R. 1998, *After Heaven: Spirituality in America Since the 1950s*, University of California Press, Berkeley.

2

The Contemporary Search for Meaning in Suffering

Maryanne Confoy

INTRODUCTION

Recently I was asked to give a talk to a group of pastoral care workers on the topic 'Spiritual Care or Pastoral Care?' My first reaction was to ask myself why there was a need for such a topic and, also, what might have been happening over the past several years as pastoral care moved from something that was an integral component of Christian ministry to a more clinical and professional identity and practice. As a consequence of my research in response to this experience, my present concern is to address the topic 'Religion, Pastoral Care, Spirituality, and the Contemporary Search for Meaning in Suffering'. I want to present some of the early sources that have influenced our understanding of pastoral care, to analyse the manner in which its early beginnings have shaped our present understanding of the term, and, subsequently, the ways in which some of the questions about pastoral care and spirituality have been affected by the changing relationship of religion and spirituality in our world today.

In those early eras, when the Christian belief system was accepted without question, the normative panorama against which questions of meaning in suffering were measured was the Christian faith, its affirmation of Jesus Christ's triumph over death, and the unquestioning belief in heaven and hell. Pastoral care was given and received in the context of this worldview. In our contemporary multifaith and secular world, questions of meaning in life in the face of suffering and death are far more complex. In responding to such questions elements of a spirituality of pastoral care are proposed.

PASTORAL CARE

The origins of words gives them a special significance, whether we are consciously aware of this or not. The term 'pastoral care' has come out of a religious context. The expression has its own history. The *Oxford English Dictionary* gives the history of the word 'pastoral'; its etymology is in its Latin origins, *pascere*—to feed. The term was first recorded in the English language in 1526—'pertaining to shepherds and their occupation' and 'pertaining to shepherds of souls; having relation to the spiritual care of a "flock" of Christians'. In an imperial world of highly respected hierarchical and honorific leadership structures, an alternative model of shepherd and sheep was chosen for the spiritual care and nourishment of the community of Christians. To understand the meaning of pastoral care we need to reflect on the community of its origins.

'Pastor' is a word that has developed within the Christian tradition and it carries its history within that tradition. Originally, the term 'pastor' was used exclusively of those ordained as ministers by their churches. In early Christianity a pastor was usually a bishop or a priest. The ordained had pastoral responsibility for the people in their care. The use of the term was varied, for example, within Roman Catholicism we read, 'Only a priest may be validly appointed pastor' (Kelly 1967, p. 1075). Also, the three 'pastoral' epistles, 1 and 2 Timothy and Titus, 'are commonly known by this term because they consist largely of instructions on Church government and discipline' (Kelly 1967, p. 1075). Such pastoral letters, written by a bishop to his flock, could be doctrinal, disciplinary, or devotional in their advice to the Christian community. This was the basic understanding of the early church and its use of the terms 'pastor' and 'pastoral'. Generated from the leadership model of the time, they indicated authority and governance in its application to the community of believers.

PASTORAL THEOLOGY

As Christendom flourished in pre-Reformation Europe the need for doctrinal orthodoxy and practical up-to-date guidelines for the exercise of pastoral ministry led to the development of pastoral theology as a separate discipline within theological studies. The classical definition of theology as 'faith seeking understanding' was that of Anselm in the twelfth century. At that time, faith simply meant the Christian faith. As Christian thinkers explored their understanding of their faith it began to be obvious that it could be subdivided into categories such as *dogmatic* or *systematic* theology, which pertained to doctrinal and moral teachings, *spiritual theology*, which focused on the inner transformation effected by the presence of grace in the human person, and *pastoral theology*, which sought to develop the implications for the actual life situation of the Church and its members, especially for ministry, preaching, and counselling. So the question about the relationship of pastoral care and spiritual care has its roots in the early dichotomy between pastoral and spiritual theology. While spiritual theology was concerned with the inner relationship between God and God's people, pastoral theology was directed towards the Church's care of the church community and its activities on behalf of the salvation of all peoples.

Pastoral theology has been consistently described as a practical science of the care of souls (Brundage 1967, p. 1080). It consisted in the application of dogmatic, moral, and spiritual theology to pastoral problems. The object of pastoral theology was to demonstrate how the various sacred sciences and related subjects could be used efficaciously for the salvation of souls. From its beginnings this care was primarily exercised through the spiritual ministration of the ordained clergy. It maintained the soul/body dualism that existed in those early and middle periods of the Church and in the society of the time.

Spiritual theology, the science of Christian perfection, was differentiated from pastoral theology by its appropriation of ascetic principles to exhort and direct those who were seen to be capable of the higher reaches of the spiritual life. New rankings of the members of the Christian community were becoming established in their efforts to strive for perfection as both monastic and apostolic religious orders of men and women were beginning to flourish. Spiritual theology was directed towards the elite Christian, while pastoral theology was for all. Questions of suffering and death were resolved by the worldview that perceived a heavenly reward or punishment as a consequence of people's life choices and the way they lived their beliefs and values.

As societies and cultures changed in the post-Reformation and modern eras, so too did the historical and geographical development of Christendom and its influence. Pastoral theologians became increasingly concerned with the developing and specific needs of the communities of their period, and the changes in the conditions and circumstances of the members of their parishes and dioceses. Change became normative. People's needs changed, social classes and structures were being redefined, and relationship patterns and work situations were in flux. Christianity's application of dogmatic and moral theology from the past needed to be addressed to new and diverse circumstances and worldviews. It was not always equal to the task.

PASTORAL AND PRACTICAL THEOLOGY

The term 'pastoral' itself has been problematic in recent eras, 'for it constantly encourages the misconception that pastoral theology is purely and simply a doctrine of the priestly office, or even that the Church's work is a matter of transitive pastoral action carried out on a passive object' (Schuster 1969, p. 365). In 1841 the term 'practical theology' was coined by the Catholic and Lutheran theological schools of Tübingen in order to address misconceptions and changing contexts of pastoral ministry that the radical cultural changes in the Western world had generated.

Perhaps one of the more important associated influences on pastoral care was the new discipline of pastoral psychology. As people became more aware of the more complex aspects of human motivation, of the inner world of people, and of the need to bring insights from the science of the inner world of the psyche, the findings of the secular discipline of psychology were introduced into the religious realm of pastoral care.

Psychology brought an alternative perspective to the task of caring in the Christian community. Consequently, theologians began to add the study of pastoral psychology to their attempts to propose pastoral principles and guidelines for authentic Christian spiritual development. Pastoral psychologists researched the essential psychological data that contributed to effective pastoral care. With these new understandings of personhood gained through psychological research, stages of religious development were gradually brought into the churches' pastoral ministry.

Pastoral psychology and pastoral care

Pastoral psychology was informed by the data accumulated in the diverse sub-disciplines within psychology to the extent to which these findings were relevant to pastoral care, but problems occurred with the selective response to and acceptance of such data by various Christian hierarchical bodies. Even in the present time there are no clearly defined limits nor any precise agreement as to what areas of psychology might furnish the most significant data for Christian pastoral care. Within Roman Catholicism, for example, goals of pastoral psychology were consonant with those of pastoral theology, particularly to aid the individual in attaining (one's) eternal salvation (cf. Biers 1967, p. 1080). However, the religious assumptions integral to a premodern period about what constitutes salvation and the question of suffering in pastoral care contexts have changed significantly in subsequent centuries.

The fundamental goal of pastoral care was to promote the wellbeing of people and to assist them in the lifelong conversion process that is integral to the Christian life. Its historical context can be clearly seen as church-based or mandated. Although originally this pastoral intent was primarily directed to the members within the Christian community, it gradually extended beyond the community to a concern for all people, especially those marginalised by illness or affliction of one sort or another. Contemporary Christian pastoral care reaches beyond the local community to the unchurched and to all who are suffering from living on the margins of church communities and/or society. From its narrower beginnings and, through the influence of Clinical Pastoral Education programs, pastoral care has gradually taken on a more professional identity, moving from the specifically clerical realm towards a more comprehensive response.

Pastoral care has been described as designating the broad range of activities carried out by ordained and nonordained ministers in response to people's needs. These activities, including sacramental and social ministries, can be as informal as conversational encounters and as formal as highly structured ritual events (Studzinski 1993, p. 722).

This expansive understanding of pastoral care has been influenced by radical changes in cultural contexts. Western culture has moved from the worldview of early Christendom to the more pragmatic restructuring of beliefs and values required by multicultural and multifaith contexts. The questioning and reshaping of our beliefs about the world and its workings have also been affected by post-Enlightenment and deconstructionist philosophies that have eroded many of the certainties that held Christian communities together in the past.

RELIGION AND SPIRITUALITY

Spirituality is now being researched in its most generic forms, both by religious believers and by people who are concerned to find transcendent meaning for their lives. Many former believers feel that their church has failed them in their times of real need. Their issue is not so much with their God, but with the ways in which the issues that preoccupy church leaders do not touch the real life pressures and problems of their church members. People are struggling to make sense of their search for meaning and purpose in their routine life situations and in the experience of suffering. When doubt is denounced by religious leaders as disloyalty or as a failure in religious ortho-doxy, people are led to repress or deny some of their foundational questions and experiences that can lead them into new depths of understanding them-selves and the mystery intrinsic to their creedal system. 'How, as an adult, do I pray to God?' 'Who is this God who allows people to die like this?' 'Where is God in my suffering?' 'How do I break through the spiritual darkness that sur-rounds me?' These are questions that pastoral care workers meet explicitly or implicitly on a daily basis. As religion in its narrow forms loses relevance for people's lives, spirituality comes into the foreground of their interests.

In its widest meaning, spirituality not only goes beyond but also includes people's beliefs, convictions, and patterns of thought, their emotions and behaviour in respect to what is ultimate, or to God. The ways people relate to each other and to their environment influence the shape their spirituality takes. Their place in society, life circumstances, the rituals and patterns of liv-ing, loving and working contribute to their spiritual development (cf. Carr 1988, p. 203). Spirituality is also shaped by the personal, familial, and cul-tural storytelling that tells us who we are and about our place in the world. When the religious story of Christianity, Judaism, Buddhism, Islam, or any religious belief system fails to intersect with the personal and communal stor-ies that confront people in the dailiness of their lives, then, that religious tradition faces its own irrelevance.

A contemporary understanding of spirituality is being sought by philoso-phers, scientists, and religious believers who are working towards a more comprehensive vision of life, its meaning, and its mystery. Diverse approaches to contemporary understandings of spirituality draw on the com-mon elements of both secular and sacred belief systems; they invite dialogue rather than dogmatism in the search for meaning and for truth. One approach to spirituality describes the human search for a unifying purpose and transcendent meaning for our lives in the pursuit of ultimate goodness. It is informed by multifaith and diverse belief perspectives and, while it has strong philosophical foundations, it remains open to new possibilities of natural or social scientific discoveries of the future. Death and suffering are not trivialised in its acknowledgment of mystery, and the significance of both individual and communal relationships are taken into account. This depiction of spirituality (which draws on Whitehead's definition of religion; cf. Whitehead 1938, pp. 191–2) shows its potential to include all aspects of our search for both an immanent and transcendent meaning for human life.

> Spirituality is forming a vision of that which stands beyond, behind, and within the passing flux of immediate things, something that is real, to be explored by a close attention to our immediate world, and yet waiting to be realised. Something that is a remote possibility and yet the greatest of present realities of our life, something that gives meaning to all that passes and yet forever eludes full apprehension, something whose possession is the ultimate good and yet as that beyond our life demands an ongoing quest, something that embeds us in relationships with others and yet at times will require a journey in solitude, a vision that makes us participants in the unfolding of the universe, yet ever mindful of and haunted by the horizon beyond that unfolding, a vision requiring the exercise of mind, heart, and body, a vision replete with consequences for action. (Anderson 2000)

One of the benefits of such an approach to spirituality is its dynamic nature. There is always a danger of closure to truth when people become embedded in a worldview, be it religious or secular.

The spiritual quest is an integral part of the human search for meaning. It has been the preoccupation of our artistic and literary endeavours throughout human history. Fuelled by our imagination and informed by religious beliefs and meaning-making systems, it has addressed the mystery of death and suffering across a range of historical and geographical cultures. Spirituality is, therefore, intimately connected to the presence or absence of 'the unquenchable fire of desire', a restlessness of the heart, a pervasive feeling of emptiness, in the lives of individuals and their communities. It is an 'all-embracing ache that lies at the centre of human experience and is the universal force that drives everything else. This dis-ease is universal. What we do with our longings, both in terms of handling the pain and the hope that they bring us, that is our spirituality' (Rolheiser 1999, pp. 4–5).

The restlessness of our hearts indicates the spiritual energy, the deep down, perhaps unheard desires that keep us from settling down to inertia or to a trivialising of our lives. Spirituality is 'more about whether or not we can sleep at night than about whether or not we go to church' (Rolheiser 1999, p. 7).

The opposite of spirituality is to be without energy or purpose in life and to have no centre of meaning or value that can give a focus to our living and loving. When human lives are without a centring focus or purpose, they dissipate energy and degenerate into addictive behaviour patterns.

Many people who have given up their religious affiliations because of their experience of disconnectedness—their dis-ease—are looking outside their churches for values and purpose. Various commentators describe the spiritual needs and interests of such groups as baby boomers, Gen X, and Gen Y seekers (Beaudoin 1999). These age cohorts share a common distrust of institutions, a suspicion of—alongside a willingness to dip into—mainstream religions and the importance of personal experience over church doctrine and ritual. They are often merged into the New Age approach to life and meaning.

> Optimism is the hallmark of the amorphous, anarchic phenomenon now known as the New Age. Its sixties style of idealism has survived both the disillusionment of the seventies and the materialism of the eighties, and shows no sign of waning. On the contrary, it has an extraordinary ability to adopt and adapt ideas from the global spiritual supermarket, and then communicate them brilliantly. It has spawned dozens of best-selling authors … In this communications revolution, through digitisation, and the Internet, everyone is empowered. As a result you no longer need the institution or church (Bunting 1998, p. 26).

Such spirituality is death denying, privatised, individualistic, and consumer-based; spiritual delights and salvation are promised with a price tag. Individuals who suffer bear the burden of New Age superficiality of beliefs, values, and meaning in the face of the ultimate mysteries of life.

SUFFERING AND PASTORAL CARE IN THE CONTEMPORARY CONTEXT

Confronted by often competing approaches to spirituality in our present society, how does the pastoral care worker address issues of meaning in suffering? With the removal of pastoral care from the religious to the public domain, how can pastoral care workers be accountable to the sometimes contradictory communities of meaning-making in which they participate? Is it possible for pastoral care workers to be attentive and responsive to their own convictions about personal faithfulness and their search for meaning in suffering as they pass through the tensions of different ages and stages in their life journey? These are important questions that pastoral care workers face in their day-by-day ministry. Perhaps it is time to revisit the early model of leadership that the founding Christian communities chose to follow.

In a Greco-Roman hierarchically structured world order, a counter-cultural model of a leader familiar with those being led was chosen. Trappings of authority were not part of such a model. Knowing and being known, companioning, and understanding were key elements of the relationship. How can such a model hold any relevance for the complex worldview and circumstances of *pastoral* care in the public domain and in the scientific technocracy in which it operates today?

TOWARDS A SPIRITUALITY OF PASTORAL CARE

Four basic activities that are integral to pastoral care fit well the pastoral aspect of ministry; together they describe a contemporary spirituality of pastoral care. These activities are guiding, sustaining, reconciling, and healing, and if each of these is taken separately then it is possible to see a ministry develop that takes account of the transformative experiences of both the minister and those being ministered to.

Guiding

In order to be authentic guides for others, pastoral carers need to be self-aware. In the past the isolated life of the shepherd meant that autonomy was an essential character trait. Self-awareness and self-understanding are dynamic rather than static features of the pastoral care worker. To be a guide is not to be a guru. New relationships and situations confront people with new insights about identity, about their beliefs and convictions and about their strengths and weaknesses in living and loving. Religious convictions can be helpful, but adherence to truths can also cause rigidity. If pastoral care workers' responses to life's questions come from outside themselves, from an unexamined acceptance of answers to life's mysteries, then they can be locked into a complacency that helps no one. To guide others, people need to have the courage to walk alone, to experience isolation, to face the dangers of questioning, of surfacing their own hopes, fears and doubts. Carers who have learnt to accept their own limitations and acknowledge their gifts are best able to companion others in their journeying.

Guiding requires the capacity to adapt to changing circumstances—their own and others. As people age and face different life and relationship issues they are called to rework their understanding of who they are in relationship to others, to God, or to what is ultimate in their lives. Carers may find that the meaning and purpose that has served them to this point now seem flat and empty. Pastoral carers may have dealt with something problematic or painful in childhood as courageously as they could have at the time, but as they age they can develop greater understanding and a greater capacity to forgive. Rather than avoid painful memories carers need to take the time to rework them and integrate them in such ways that they can free themselves from self-images or patterns of behaving from the past that are no longer authentic and that inhibit their capacity to companion others on their journey. Guides need to accompany others on their journeys. People's faith or doubts may not be those of carers, who need to be attentive to where they are in their own human journey and where they may be called to follow as companions.

Sustaining

Pastoral care requires steadfastness of presence. This type of ministry requires people to be present through the long haul of healing and across a range of experiences of suffering and care. 'It seems to me that the minister must be prepared not to fall back on traditional forms but to try simply *to be there*, to show ... solidarity with [people] in [their] sickness' (Faber 1971, p. 51). It is not enough to go through the appearance—or even a sacramental ritual—of caring; carers need to have an authentic presence to those they are visiting or supporting. This requires not only the vulnerability of the wounded healer, but also the presence of a person with strong beliefs and convictions.

To sustain others in their experiences of suffering and loss pastoral care workers need to have firm foundations and support systems themselves. No one can keep offering spiritual support and nourishment to others unless their own supply is being replenished. Times of care for others need to be balanced by times of self-care. To be authentic during times of conversation with those in need and with other pastoral carers requires the ability to be still, to be able to take time for contemplation, to be in touch with one's own inner thoughts, feelings, and imaginative awareness. Times of prayerful support of others call for times of inner quiet and solitude.

Experiences of separation and connectedness are constantly present to the pastoral care worker. People move in and out of the world of pastoral carers.

While the ability to be present to others—that is, the carer joins with the other in his or her suffering and does not remain at a self-protective distance—is important, carers must be able to let go when the time comes. The connectedness comes at a price, which can sometimes be quite unexpected and unusual. When pastoral carers are present to other people's suffering, their presence may be experienced tangibly. The report of a woman visitor who became violently ill while she was sitting with a terminally ill friend showed that she had picked up the pain of her friend. Such anecdotes illustrate the ways in which empathy in its most intense form can cause suffering to the carer as well as to the one in pain. Without realising it pastoral carers can, on occasions, become quite debilitated because they are carrying the sufferings of others within themselves (cf. Fiand 1999, pp. 95–101). Tensions of separation and connectedness call for a high degree of self-awareness in carers.

Another aspect of sustaining self in experiences of connectedness and separation is in relation to times of transition within the individual's own life journey. The initial support system and structures set up by pastoral carers will usually need to be reviewed after several years of active engagement in ministry. Carers may find themselves confronted by experiences of uneasiness, rising levels of anger or frustration with themselves, or with the institution in which they are working. Their relationships with significant others may come into question. Past feelings of affirmation and purpose in ministry may be replaced by new questions, fears, and anxieties. Whether to allow these to surface can be a further problem to those whose outer world takes precedence over their inner world. Past resolutions of belief or unbelief come under threat, or call for revision.

These transitional periods can recur on a regular basis every several years. Rather than see them as times of failure in faith or ministry, pastoral care workers may recognise these unsettling periods as opportunities for new growth. Relationship networks and priorities also call for regular revision over the years. Carers can integrate aspects of their living, loving, and serving others that may have changed or require reworking in terms of the learning provided by the decade or so of experience that is theirs.

Reconciling

To be reconciled requires the ability to stand apart, to take counsel, again and again. The roots of the word indicate a process of deliberation, a context of both giving and receiving advice, and the experience of gathering together to deliberate. So both individual and communal processes are integral to reconciliation. Pastoral care workers are called on to take counsel over and over. Their ministry usually requires them to function in a community of communities. Within the healthcare context they attend to the concerns of the person who asks for their support, to clinicians—medical and nursing staff—who are treating the person, to those who visit and care for the person. Taking counsel in this context means that pastoral carers need to know when and how to share the counsel received and when to keep silence.

To be a pastoral care worker is usually to be a member of a team, with all the strengths and weaknesses of the team identity. If a hospital is to be a place of 'hospitality' rather than 'a factory in which only efficiency and production-figures are of importance, then we must grasp firmly that only a team of people, each as an expert with (their) own task to do, yet able *as a people* to carry responsibility, can make a hospital into a community of human beings' (Faber 1971, p. 69). Where pressures of working in the context of suffering and possible death are constantly confronted, people need to be collaborators whose respect for each other's profession stands without question.

Reconciliation calls for time and energy to be given to meeting times so that team workers can listen to each other and hear the diverse perspectives that are brought to service, healing, and ministry. Team work is characterised by authentic dialogue, in which people listen to each other with faith, hope, trust, and critical self-awareness, and where conflict is addressed rather than escaped from. This is in contrast to monological encounters and conversational pleasantries from which there can be no growth because there is no real exchange of ideas or interests. Dialogue also requires recognition that the person suffering needs to be part of the team. People who face their own experiences of loss, of raw pain, and radical reviewing of their lives can contribute to the lives of those with whom they come into contact. Vulnerability brings out the best and the worst in human beings; the pastoral care worker has the opportunity—and, perhaps, the responsibility—to reconcile these elements. Compassionate caring can help people to embrace their limits as well as their strengths.

After a decade or so of ministry it is not unusual for carers to find themselves facing symptoms of depression and/or darkness. These painful symptoms of inner suffering call for new levels of reconciliation within carers themselves. Negative feelings can be attended to, or they can be repressed. Carers who respond with rejection of, or rigidity to, their own inner voices have little to offer those who are facing life's ultimate questions.

The consequence of denial is loss of energy and purpose, and the pervasive feeling of both tiredness and loss of direction and meaning for life. To the extent that they take time to do their inner work, pastoral care workers may find that they are growing in greater self-understanding and have new levels of freedom in their ministry. Their relationship with their God, or their understanding of what is of ultimate value in their lives may be reworked and revisioned, thereby enabling them to become sources of strength to those with whom they communicate their care.

Healing

Multiple levels of healing are operative in any situation of suffering or illness. The physical level of healing is the most obvious. Yet the healthcare system has changed over the years so that the original aspect of 'hospitality' that was integral to the term 'hospital' has changed radically. A new environment has been established in which patients have become clients and 'repair' and 'replacement' have become operative terms for the healing process. This has positive and negative aspects. The ministry of the pastoral carer intersects with all the varied interests of those engaged in a healthcare institution. In such a setting, physical healing is normally of primary importance, and the operative understanding of the meaning of life and death has a major impact on the ethos of a hospital, its personnel, and its activities. Acceptance of the inevitability of death in previous eras has been replaced by the contemporary effort to conquer it—or at least postpone it as long as possible.

Hospitals are places 'where the battle against death is most fiercely fought, often to the bitter end. It is part of the creed of the medical and nursing staff that death can never be accepted, and many patients find themselves caught up in this stand (Faber 1971, p. 56). This comment is still true in those healthcare settings where the mechanisation of dying prevails. Pastoral care workers may find themselves facing the same dilemma as that faced by the brother of a dying woman in an intensive care ward where machines and tubes took control. 'I would have liked to hold her hand, or when she became restless, to wipe the sweat off her forehead. But it was impossible. I caught myself behaving very differently than I intended. I was changed from being a brother, who wanted to be with his dying sister, into a component of the dying-machine to which she was attached' (Sölle 1999, p. 80). All those involved in the clinical process are doing the best they can for the suffering individual, but they can be working from competing and sometimes conflicting approaches to suffering and healing. A contemporary attitude to the question of suffering that moves away from religious explanations and takes the greater complexity of technological context and clinical perspectives into account is described by Per Anderson. He points out that the forms suffering takes 'are also the stuff of cultural systems. Humans never suffer radically alone. Moments of self-conflict and refusal are conditioned by the socially grounded interpretive apparatus we bring to experience. In this way, the "problem of suffering", like the particular response it elicits, should be understood as a cultural form' (Anderson, in Mohrmann & Hanson (eds) 1999, p. 130). For the pastoral worker, today's cultural form of suffering has to be respected, but it cannot violate the person's own understanding of suffering and its mystery. Technology's promise to remove suffering from people's experience has not been substantiated by its results to date (cf. Anderson 1999, p. 126). Healing can take place in time of great suffering and, while physical healing may be real, inner suffering may be debilitating to an individual.

Within the medical profession a more holistic approach to suffering and to healing is being taken into account. Clinicians such as Benson (1996) and Siegel (1986) have taken the mind/body/belief system into their clinical response. New disciplines such as psychooncology and psychoneuroimmunology are moving into the clinical conversation. The physiological and spiritual mysteries of mind/body healing are the subject of an increasing amount of medical dialogue and research.

Spiritual writer Henri Nouwen's notion of the 'wounded healer' has been significant for many engaged in peoplework over the years. It is difficult for those involved in pastoral care, especially those who have been trained in theological schools, or who are professional or ordained ministers, to be present to the questions, fears, and doubts of others when they are going through the same type of questioning themselves. It is not uncommon for some involved in pastoral care to appear to lose their faith. What they may have lost is the faith of easy answers, the faith of religious ideology, or the faith that is exclusive and judgmental in its approach to suffering.

Sometimes individuals can go through periods of atheism or agnosticism when they are confronted by the horrific sufferings of others, the tragedy of a child's death, or the impact on people and their carers of demeaning and protracted illnesses such as Alzheimer's disease and other forms of dementia. Such individuals may move from a former comfortable certainty of believing in a God who punishes the evil and rewards the good, to the realisation that life is mystery and that all attempts to know God are limited by our human finiteness. Suffering constantly confronts believers with the limits of their understanding of an unconditionally loving God. A period of great spiritual emptiness may be the forerunner of a new leap of faith, hope, and love that transforms people's earlier and more simplistic forms of believing and loving God. When pastoral carers are able to let go of their own constructions of God, and when they realise that they cannot control their own lives—let alone the lives of others—then they are moving into a deeper awareness of their identity as wounded healers.

Nouwen did not describe a healer whose scar has replaced the wound. To care authentically for others—and for oneself—is to be open to suffering, to being wounded on behalf of others, and to the lifelong need for healing. Sometimes this healing can take the shape of a healing of our personal memories. Perhaps someone else's experience may be a catalyst for the recalling of an experience of unresolved pain in our own past. Or what may come to the surface of our consciousness may be a healing of our family or our society's collective memory. We are all wounded by our past and need to be healed from those wounds. We all also need to be healed from the wounds we have inflicted on our companions. Awareness of this brings a deeper sensibility to the multilevelled experiences of healing and being healed. Compassion is the fruit of such healing experiences.

CONCLUSION

Pastoral care has moved a long way from its earliest origins in Christendom. It has been removed from the context of a single religious worldview to a world where a multiplicity of religious and secular belief systems contribute to the human understanding of meaning and purpose for life in the face of suffering and death. The original choice of a counter-cultural model of leadership remains significant for our present time. Pastoral care calls for transformation of all those involved in care—whether they are professionals in the field, or those receiving care. The contemporary understanding of an inclusive spirituality informs personal and communal beliefs and values. It also includes people's lifelong striving for meaning in a world that maintains its mystery alongside its moments of revelation. The spirituality of pastoral workers is directed towards their own lifelong affirmation of the fullness of living and loving in face of the mystery of suffering and death.

REFERENCES

Anderson, P. 1999, 'To change and to accept in a technological society', in M. E. Mohrmann & M. J. Hanson (eds), *Pain Seeking Understanding: Suffering, Medicine and Faith*, The Pilgrim Press, Cleveland, pp. 126, 130.

Anderson, R. 2000, <http://www2.bc.edu/~anderso/sr/spirituality.html>. Accessed July 2000.

Beaudoin, T. 1999 'GenX spirituality', *TIKKUN*, vol. 13, no. 5, pp. 45, 67.

Benson, H. 1996, *Timeless Healing: The Power and Biology of Belief*, Scribner, New York.

Bier, W. C. 1967, 'Pastoral psychology', *New Catholic Encyclopedia*, vol. 10, Catholic University of America, Washington, DC, pp. 1078–80.

Brundage, J. A. 1967, 'Pastoral theology', *New Catholic Encyclopedia*, vol. 10, Catholic University of America, Washington, DC, pp. 1080–84.

Bunting, M. 1998, 'Coming of Age', *Guardian Weekly*, London, vol. 159, issue 16, 18 October, p. 26.

Carr, A. 1988, *Transforming Grace*, Harper & Row, San Francisco, p. 203.

Faber, H. 1971, *Pastoral Care in the Modern Hospital*, trans. Hugo de Waal, Westminster Press, Philadelphia, pp. 51, 56, 59.

Fiand, B. 1999, *Prayer and the Quest for Healing: Our Personal Transformation and Cosmic Responsibility*, Crossroad, New York, pp. 95–101.

Kelly, B. 1967, 'Pastor', *New Catholic Encyclopedia*, vol. 10, Catholic University of America, Washington, DC, pp. 1075–76.

Rahner, K. (ed.) 1969, *Sacramentum Mundi: An Encyclopedia of Theology*, Herder & Herder, New York, vol. IV.

Rolheiser, R. 1999, *The Holy Longing: The Search for a Christian Spirituality*, Doubleday, New York, pp. 4–5.

Schuster, H. 1969 'Pastoral Theology' in K. Rahner (ed.), *Sacramentum Mundi: An Encyclopedia of Theology*, Herder & Herder, New York, vol. Ivb, pp. 365–8.

Siegel, B. 1986, *Love, Medicine and Miracles*, Harper & Row, New York.

Sölle, D. 1999, *Against the Wind: Memoir of a Radical Christian*, Augsburg, Minneapolis, p. 80.

Studzinski, R. 1993, 'Pastoral care and counseling', in M. Downey (ed.), *The New Dictionary of Catholic Spirituality*, Liturgical Press, Collegeville, Minnesota, p. 722.

Whitehead, A. N. 1938, *Science and the Modern World*, Penguin, Harmondsworth, pp. 191–2.

3

Towards a Philosophy of Caring and Spirituality for a Secular Age

Stan van Hooft

INTRODUCTION

Spirituality is a minor theme in the literature of medicine, nursing, and other healthcare professions. When it does occur, numerous philosophical questions are raised. Many texts stress the need for the clinician to take the religious beliefs and needs of patients into account and to accord them proper respect. But they do so without challenging the spiritual perspectives of the clinicians themselves. The position of such texts is that the spirituality of the patient is an aspect of the problem with which the clinician has to deal, an aspect that can have a negative or positive impact upon the clinical treatment depending upon how it is handled. Some patients will fail to cooperate with treatment because of their religious convictions, while others will find comfort and encouragement in their beliefs. But for the clinician, the appropriate stance is one of objectivity and detachment tempered by respect and tolerance (Waldfogel 1997). Other texts urge a growth in spiritual awareness or a spiritual renewal in healthcare practitioners themselves on the grounds that the kinds of spiritual support that patients need can only be given by practitioners who are deeply imbued with such convictions (Gaut & Boykin 1994; Stoter 1998). Other texts (Hafen et al. 1996; Epperly 1997) describe the 'the healing power of spirituality' and the essential place of spiritual fulfilment in our concept of health.

But the philosophical problem on which I want to concentrate is that of understanding what spirituality is in the context of healthcare generally and in the context of palliative care more specifically. Once we have understood this, the issue of whether care-givers need to have a spiritual life of their own in order to be effective will resolve itself.

Many texts that discuss spirituality in healthcare assume that there is an intrinsic connection between spirituality on the one hand, and metaphysics and religion on the other. For example, one text summarises research into healthcare practitioners' perceptions of what spiritual health is by listing the following features:

- something that gives meaning or purpose to life
- a set of principles or ethics to live by
- the sense of selflessness and a feeling for others—a willingness to do more for others than for yourself
- commitment to God and an ultimate concern
- perception of what causes the universe to work the way it does
- something for which there is no rational explanation—recognition of powers beyond the natural and rational
- something perceived as being known or hazily known—something for which there is no easy explanation, and so becomes a matter of faith
- the most pleasure-producing quality of humans (Hafen et al. 1996, p. 380).

This is a broad list, one that includes religion, morality, cosmology, mysticism, a sense of self-worth, the feeling that life is worth living, and that rather puzzling reference to pleasure. I offer it here not only because it illustrates the frequent link between spirituality and belief in a transcendent reality, but also because it indicates what a wide range of concerns and questions can be embraced by the concept of the spiritual. It will require some philosophical reflection to see whether there is any connection between the various issues that are raised in this list and whether belief in a reality beyond that of this world is central to them in any way.

SPIRITUALITY AND METAPHYSICS

The most significant thinker in the Western philosophical tradition to give expression to such the questions already raised in this chapter was Plato. Most broadly and most simply put, Plato suggested that our worldly existence and the material world in which we play it out are but shadowy copies of a more perfect order of reality in which everything is as it should be and in which the ideals of goodness, beauty, and truth could be directly apprehended by souls that were relatively free from their earthly existence. It seemed inconceivable to Plato, and to many of his educated followers, including Aristotle, that the world that they saw around them and the mode of existence which they experienced within themselves should be the source of ultimate meaning for life. The world was too full of change. Knowledge of it was too uncertain. Human existence was too fragile. Human aspirations were too ensnared in emotion and desire. How could a world that was full of danger and unpredictability be the proper object of human reason and contemplation? How could human life be meaningful if all it contained was the more or less successful pursuit of biological needs and a mélange of disreputable passions? Surely human beings were possessed of an immortal soul by virtue of which they participated in the life of the gods and through which they had access to a higher order of reality? It seemed obvious that worldly, everyday existence was unworthy of the humanity that had been bestowed upon us.

Notice that this conception of human life assumes the existence of a realm of transcendence. Before even postulating it as a philosophical or theological system, Plato adopted the ancient Greek conception of an order of reality in which fate ensured that all things transpired as they were destined to do and where justice ruled as an objective and purposive force ensuring the balance of good and evil in the cosmos (Cornford 1912). Even today, when, for example, we consider it unfair that a person of achievement and virtue should be struck down prematurely by a fatal illness, we are expressing this ancient faith in a cosmic order that will ensure the rightness of what luck has made inevitable.

Plato was too good a philosopher to allow this deeply held assumption of the justice of fate to serve as a premise for an argument. After all, what right do we have to simply assume that the blind, causal processes of nature should produce outcomes that are fair? His conviction that a realm of perfection existed and that it influenced our lives was built on arguments that have continued to influence thinkers through the ages. He postulated a realm of 'Forms', which enjoyed the theoretical necessity of *a priori* reason. It would be impossible, Plato reasoned, to see things as equal if we did not believe in Absolute Equality, and it would be impossible to experience beauty if we did not have a way of apprehending Absolute Beauty. Moreover, things could not be what they were if there were not an Essence that accounted for their being definitely that and not something else. Knowledge of these essences would not only allow us to apprehend things correctly so as to bring us into contact with Truth, but would also bring us under the influence of the eternal realm of forms to which they belonged and thereby make us virtuous.

For Plato, virtuous human beings were those who could overcome the desires that would beguile their bodies and tie them to their earthly existence so as to set the intellectual life of the soul free to be influenced by pure knowledge of the Form of Goodness. It is clear to anyone who thinks about it that we are not just creatures of desire. However, important as our desires and enthusiasms might be in giving zest to our lives, they do not give it a point. The satisfaction of our desires—when fate allows it to us—does not ultimately satisfy. We simply go on to desire more. Moreover, it is clear that our reason is not just in the service of our desires. While it is true that we human beings have tremendous abilities in thinking strategically with a view to fulfilling our needs and wishes, this is not the only form that our thinking takes. Our effectiveness today in colonising the entire earth and our efficiency in producing technologies that reduce work to little more than scheduling the use of sophisticated tools are evidence of immense rational powers. But should efficiency be the sole goal of these powers?

Plato argued that the fundamentally important role for these powers was *theoria*. By this he meant the arts of contemplation, reflection, and theorising. For his part, Aristotle distinguished between a 'calculative part of the soul' and a 'contemplative part of the soul'. The first represented those functions of reason that were exercised in the practical, everyday affairs of human beings, while the second represented those functions exercised when human beings turn their minds to eternal and changeless things. In today's terms the disciplines that embody this latter form of rationality are pure mathematics, theoretical physics, astronomy, philosophy, theology, and conceptual art. These forms of thinking are useless in terms of our material needs, but they do represent a human tendency for thought that reaches beyond the everyday necessities of life towards the whole of reality and towards the depths of reality's meanings.

Plato and Aristotle argued that human beings are possessed of this contemplative form of reason by relying on a remarkable premise: namely, that transcendent objects must have a human faculty corresponding to them. If there are purely theoretical objects for us to think about then we must have the ability to think in purely theoretical terms. Just as the Pythagoreans who inspired Plato had thought that numbers were real, so Plato thought that whatever abstractions our theoretical reason could conceive must also be real. If these Forms are real, then we must be possessed of a spiritual soul to be the faculty for contemplating these realities. And so was born the spiritual life of the Western intellectual and metaphysical tradition.

It is now well known how this philosophy became absorbed into the mainstream of Western religion. Struggling to give expression to the salvific message of Jesus in philosophically sophisticated terms, the Greek-speaking fathers of the early Christian church used Plato to replace the immanent personal God of the Hebrews with a transcendent, providential, and universal Form of Goodness. Later, using the concepts of Aristotle, they turned that god into a prime mover and cause of all things. For its part, the soul was no longer the function of being alive, of having desires, of being intelligent, and of reaching towards the transcendent, but an immortal, spiritual entity, the fate of which became the Christian's primary concern in life. Theology became the expression of theoretical reason whose task it was to use the constructions of philosophy to give rational coherence to the content of faith. But the fundamental terms of such constructions had been set before the gospel message was heard. These constructions presupposed a profound distinction between this unworthy world and the realm of supernatural perfection. The transcendent realm was everything this world was not and everything that we, of this world, hankered after. Despite the message of the incarnation, the divide between this world and the transcendent realm was reinforced by theology and the distance between them became increasingly unbridgeable. God was conceived as a providential agency existing outside of his creation. Kant might be said to represent the high point of this transcendentalist tendency. For him, God and other metaphysical conceptions, such as our own free will, were concepts that were beyond our understanding and that belonged to a realm of noumenal reality that could not be grasped by us in knowledge. We may achieve vague intimations of these ideas of reason through the experience of beauty in art, but no direct knowledge of these transcendent realities was available to merely mortal, rational beings.

If Plato had given us any indication as to how the two realms of being might be bridged it was his strikingly spiritualised conception of love. Plato's notion of *eros* was the notion of an inherent human longing for the transcendent, a longing that is elicited by beautiful persons but comes to full fruition only in the utter rejection of any worldly involvements and attachments. The notion of the spiritual life that emerges from this conception is that of longing for the unattainably transcendent, contemplation of the theoretical, abstract, and changeless laws of reality, faith in the objectivity of Goodness, Beauty, and Truth, and knowledge, which is fulfilled in thought rather than action.

But this Platonic form of spirituality, which Western thought and religion has inherited, might well rest on a mistake. It rests on the argument that it is the existence of transcendent objects that necessitates our having a faculty for contemplating those objects. According to the arguments in the *Phaedo*, the soul must be the immortal organ for transcendent knowledge because the objects of such knowledge are themselves immortal and eternal. In Aristotle's more worldly conception, human happiness could only be achieved through the fulfilment of our faculties. The soul was possessed of a part that was the faculty of contemplation because, in a world with a transcendent dimension, there could be no fulfilment without such contemplation. The objective reality of the transcendent realm of eternal things required our possession of a contemplative soul so as to enable us to participate in the life of the gods and thereby achieve the highest form of human happiness.

SPIRITUALITY IN MODERN PHILOSOPHY

Beginning with Descartes, modern philosophy, in contrast, focused upon the subject. Rather than beginning with a worldview in which the objective reality of the transcendent realm was assumed, it began with the indubitability of subjective experience and derived the reality of God and other metaphysical conceptions from that. The culmination of this tendency was seen in Kant, whose vast philosophical achievements lay in the analysis of how the rational intellect could assure itself of the objectivity of its knowledge. And yet, for Kant, the reality of the transcendent could be accepted only on the basis of a rationally justified assumption. In the view of modern philosophy, the reality of the spiritual or contemplative functions of our minds does not rest on the actuality of the transcendent but on a reflective awareness of ourselves as thinking beings; as a result, the objective warrantability of beliefs in transcendent realities became problematic. There would always be a suspicion that belief in the metaphysical beings central to the spiritual life was a mere projection of the yearnings of human subjects.

Philosophy and theology would still be grappling with proofs for the existence of God, for theoretical foundations for universal moral standards, for objective criteria for beauty, and for quasimathematical proofs in science if it were not for the question posed by Nietzsche: 'What, really, is it in us that wants "the truth"? … Why not rather untruth?' (Nietzsche 1973). Nietzsche's challenging suggestion is that philosophy consists in our telling ourselves stories so that we can face up to the challenges of life and hide the most fundamental motivations that ground our being. Whether these stories are true is of no consequence. Can the purposes of a spiritual, contemplative life be served even if the content of the beliefs central to that life were not objective realities? Can we be ethical without believing in objective and universal moral principles? Can we be religious in the sense of having an ultimate concern without believing in God? Can we be moved by the beauty of nature without believing that nature participates in objective Beauty? Can we develop technologies without having a scientific theory of everything? Do we need a conviction that the contents of our beliefs are objective realities in order to have a spiritual life? Perhaps what the existence in our lives of a contemplative faculty, or a theoretical form of reason, or a yearning for the transcendent, tells us is not that there is a spiritual reality out there to accord with these subjective modes of being, but that these modes of being are important in themselves.

Nietzsche declared that human beings need what was later to be called a 'grand narrative' in order to place themselves into a context that would give their vulnerable lives a meaning. Even Socrates, in the *Phaedo*, had admitted that the proofs for the immortality of the soul that he had developed were little more than a means for encouraging the self in the face of death. And Kant's 'proof' for the existence of God was that we needed such a postulate in order to give point to the project of being moral.

So is our spiritual life a sham? A mere fiction created for self-encouragement? The self-defeating subjective postulation of an objective guarantor of our knowledge and values? Are we actually little more than biologically sophisticated animals pursuing our useless desires until we suffer a meaningless death? What can we find within our subjectivity that would give point to the burdens of life?

What we are left with in our postmodern, secular age is a focus on subjectivity that accords no importance to the objective truth upon which we direct our spiritual attention. If Descartes had needed a divine guarantor for the truth of our knowledge, the postmodern thinker is satisfied with pragmatic criteria for truth (Rorty 1979). In this conception the world does not need a metaphysical counterpart of perfection to give substance to its truth claims or objectivity to its values. Even in religious thought, Kierkegaard has shown that it is the subjectivity of faith rather than its concordance with objective truth that grounds the salvific efficacy of belief. And so the task of philosophy has changed. It is no longer that of establishing the objectivity of knowledge and values, but of exploring subjectivity as the ground of knowledge, morality, and spirituality.

SPIRITUALITY AND SUBJECTIVITY

In the contemporary world spirituality as a personal quest for meaning is to be sought in worldly existence rather than beyond it. Even more radically, it is to be sought within subjectivity rather than outside of oneself. Rather than attaching oneself to an objective reality—transcendent or otherwise—postmodern spirituality seeks meaning within the self. But what prevents this search from being a form of self-indulgence and a self-centred turning away from worldly engagement? What prevents it from becoming an elevation of the self into the stature of a being of transcendent importance? How can we avoid the hubris of making ourselves into gods?

The antidote to such existential self-aggrandisement is honesty. What we will find when we pursue the path to subjectivity in depth is not some deep-seated contact with a transcendent reality or a basis for spiritual self-assurance, but an all too human mélange of fear, desire, self-assertion, and longing. Even Plato could see that the love which drove us to seek Beauty, Truth, and Goodness was driven by a sense of lack within ourselves. For his part, Nietzsche spoke of the will to power as a drive towards self-affirmation and competitiveness, a drive that expressed itself in the highest achievements of art and philosophy. Modern thought has seen a proliferation of theories that disabuse humanity of its transcendentalist pretensions. Freud postulated sexuality as the basic drive behind culture and religion. Marx explained even the most noble expressions of philosophy and theology as being so much ideological superstructure hiding the self-seeking of economic class warfare. The sociobiological writers hypothesised a selfish genetic basis to even our most moral behaviour patterns and spiritual modes of thought. And Zygmunt Bauman has argued that it is fear of death that lies at the foundation of our spiritual quest. Given our vulnerability and our inevitable deaths, we seek immortality in the achievements of our families, our nations, our cultures, and our histories. While our own lives are short, our deeds and attachments will live after us, whether in the form of future generations or in the form of our own accomplishments in the world (Bauman 1992).

If the subjective search for spirituality was seen in ancient philosophy as a response to the assumed existence of a transcendent reality, and by modern philosophy as a response to the threatening possibility that this reality was a mere projection of human desire, the postmodern search acknowledges itself as a response to human vulnerability. It is this that makes the self-aggrandising turn inwards and become self-defeating. We do not find within ourselves the strength or wholeness that would be needed to ground a spiritual life. Within ourselves we find only uncertainty, vulnerability, and mortality.

THE SIGNIFICANCE OF DEATH

What is impressive about Bauman's thesis is that it places our mortality at the centre of the problem of what drives our spiritual quest. It is worth remembering that the proofs for the immortality of the soul offered by Socrates, which make such essential use of Plato's theory of Forms, are offered on the eve of Socrates' judicial execution as a form of consolation to his friends and as a justification of the spiritual quest that is the philosophical life. It is death that provides the horizon of urgency for this entire dialogue and, I suggest, for the ideas presented in it.

It is also death that provides the horizon of finitude to the conception of human existence developed by Martin Heidegger in his *Being and Time* (Heidegger 1996). In that great work human existence is conceived as an immanent being-within-the-world and being-with-others, which gains its ethical character from the 'resoluteness' of the way it faces death. If subjectivity were seen as concern for its own existence and as a grasping of its own possibilities, then death would be seen as the final negation of such grasping and concern. But for all its orientation towards the future and its possibilities, subjectivity must embrace that most final of all of its possibilities. So death must not be seen as a negation of meaning but as its necessary horizon. What would be the nature of a spiritual life lived without a transcendental dimension because the possibility of a self-transcending, timeless creation of values is cut off by death? For Heidegger, at this stage of his thinking, such a spiritual life consisted in the pursuit of authenticity in the face of the inevitable end that our lives had in store.

But there are other options. Even if philosophy no longer endorses a mode of self-transcendence that would take us towards an objective and metaphysical realm of meaning, whether it be the Good or God, it can speak of a mode of self-transcendence that takes us towards mystery and mystical union with that which is other than ourselves. We can break out of the circle of subjectivity and that which subjectivity constitutes as its own creation. We need not be confined to a world grasped by us in forms constituted by our own knowledge. We can have a spiritual dimension to our lives by reaching out to a form of mystery and infinity that is not metaphysical in nature and yet not the creation of our own subjectivity. This mystery is that of other subjectivities which I encounter in interpersonal relationships.

THE SPIRITUALITY OF THE 'OTHER'

Emmanuel Levinas has theorised this form of encounter in a remarkable analysis of what it is to gaze into the face of another person (Levinas 1961, pp. 194ff.). The eyes of the other with whom I am in encounter are looking out at me. They do not just disclose the depth and ungraspability of the personality of the other. They also disclose the mystery of the subjectivity of the other. Whence is this looking which I apprehend? Levinas speaks of the infinity of the other. The significance of the notion of 'infinity' here is not that of the mathematically limitless, but of the unplumbable depth of the personhood of the other. The significance of the notion of 'the other' is that there is no conceptual scheme or form of knowledge that will bring this other into my world. It is sheer 'alterity'. It is never going to be appropriated by me in the way that things in the world can be as an item available to me for my use. If knowledge is a form of appropriation of the world, then no knowledge of the other is possible. It is for this reason that apprehension of the other is a mystical experience. It establishes rapport with infinity. It is an encounter with mystery.

Moreover, it requires a stance that is fundamentally ethical. It is always open to me to relate to another as to an item in *my* world. Just as a piece of equipment is an item in *my* world when I use it and potentially mine when I do not, so the other person with whom I have a casual and pragmatic relationship—whether she be a bus driver, a secretary, or a colleague—can be an item in my world. Such a functional structuring of the other is a denial of their mystery and requires a blindness to their infinity. It is an appropriation of them just in their pragmatic dimension. An ethical stance towards the other, on the other hand, acknowledges the limitless breadth of the other and lets them be in their mystery. The gaze into the eyes of that other is the occasion which elicits that ethical response because it cannot but disclose the infinity of the other. It is the very ontological nature of the other as infinite mystery that constitutes the form of apprehension of that other as ethical rather than cognitive.

Being ethical rather than cognitive means that the response to the other is practical rather than contemplative. Apprehending another person as 'other' is not an exercise of theoretical reason or contemplative thought. It is the taking of a practical stance. It is a letting the other be and it is a making oneself available to that other. I do not mean by this only that I am available to the other in their need. While this might be the case and might be an appropriate response to the other when they are in fact in need, Levinas's conception is of an ethical stance that precedes any assessment of need. The primordial, ethical stance is not just a tendering of help when it is needed; it is the acknowledgment of a reality that is beyond my own. It is the recognition of a subjectivity that is transcendent to my own and yet not a threat to me. I must not appropriate the other.

What is the nature of this primordial, ethical rapport that is ontologically established as a fundamental form of my awareness of the other? If Heidegger had suggested that my fundamental relationship to my own subjectivity is one of care and concern, Levinas suggests that such care and concern are also extended to the other. The fundamental orientation of a sensitive subject towards the other is that of caring. While this might sound like little more than an elaboration of the point that the encounter with the other is a call to ethics, it has a more profound meaning. The other is a mystery with whom one enters into a mystical rapport. This is constitutive of a nonmetaphysical spirituality. As such, the rapport sets up a relationship of love in Plato's sense of a spiritual yearning. One cares for the other with whom one is in interpersonal encounter because one recognises in the other the infinity of subjectivity that is oneself. One cares for the other into whose face one is gazing because one recognises there the depth and mystery out of which one's own subjectivity is reaching towards that other. Moreover, one recognises there the vulnerability that one feels oneself. One feels there the mortality and fear of annihilation that one senses within oneself. One cannot but care for this mystery that is an echo of one's own.

If Plato had argued that the objective and transcendent reality of the Form of Goodness elicits my virtuous response, Levinas argues that it is the other who does so. 'The being that expresses itself imposes itself, but does so precisely by appealing to me with its destitution and nudity—its hunger—without my being able to be deaf to that appeal. Thus in expression the being that imposes itself does not limit but promotes my freedom, by arousing my goodness' (Levinas 1961, p. 200).

If the vulnerability of the other can elicit my caring and virtuous response to the other's mystery, then we have here the basis of a nonmetaphysical spirituality that is yet a transcending of self-concern.

SPIRITUALITY AND CARING

On this conception, caring for the other is more than a tending to the other in his or her need. It is a fundamental ontological relationship between two subjectivities. A subjectivity cannot be apprehended as an object. Our own fundamental nature as a striving-to-be apprehends worldly things merely as objects that might be of use. In this sense Plato was right: the world is not worthy of our highest contemplation. But our own fundamental nature as a striving-to-be apprehends an other in an ethical letting-that-other-be. This is a form of rapport that acknowledges the infinite worth of the other and echoes that contemplative form of thought that the ancients thought would be elicited by the eternal and perfect objects of thought which existed in a transcendental realm. Just as it was love as *eros* that was the appropriate stance towards this metaphysical reality, so the appropriate quality of our rapport with the other is that of caring.

Such caring is especially apposite in the context of healthcare generally and palliative care more specifically. Professional carers in these fields confront patients who are in the most dire need. Illness, injury, disability, and other forms of dysfunction create in their victims a condition of need that should elicit from anyone a solicitous response and a willingness to help. In the case of patients close to death, the need is even greater, not just for physical palliation and comfort, but also for spiritual assistance and support. The caring that is called for in these situations is the professional responsibility of care-givers in a variety of fields such as medicine, nursing, chaplaincy, and counselling. But such caring can be consistent with the objectification of the person who is in need. The caring to which Levinas's thinking points is of a deeper nature. It is not just a virtuous disposition or a generous professional stance. It is a fundamental ontological structure of the subjectivity that enters into encounter with the other. Such caring is not just the practical response of tendering help to those in need of it, though it may be the deep basis for such a response. Rather, the ontological kind of caring that Levinas is pointing towards is a spiritual orientation of the self that acknowledges the other in his or her mystery.

Insofar as I mirror myself in that mystery, this deep form of caring is also an acknowledgment of the vulnerability, the finitude, and the mortality of the other. Whatever be the need that others are subject to at particular junctures of their lives, their mystery and infinity are always circumscribed by the mortality, physicality, and contingency that I too am subject to. Rather than reaching out to a metaphysical realm of certainty and solace, I reach out to others in their shared vulnerability.

We are but subjectivities and we cannot make ourselves into certainties or gods. Our spiritual life is a life of rapport and encounter within a contingent world that we cannot control. If there is a transcendence available to us in this world it is to be found in the mystery of the other. If there is a spirituality available to us in this world it is to be found in the infinite depth of the other. If there is consolation available to us in this world it is to be found in the mutuality of encounter between vulnerable and mortal beings.

REFERENCES

Bauman, Z. 1992, *Mortality, Immortality and Other Life Strategies*, Polity Press, Cambridge.

Cornford, F. M. 1912, *From Religion to Philosophy: A Study in the Origins of Western Speculation*, Harper & Row, New York.

Epperly, B. G. 1997, *Spirituality & Health: Health & Spirituality*, Twenty-Third Publications, Mystic, Connecticut.

Gaut, D. A. & Boykin, A. (eds) 1994, *Caring as Healing: Renewal Through Hope*, National League for Nursing Press, New York.

Hafen, B. Q. et al. 1996, *Mind/Body Health: The Effects of Attitudes, Emotions and Relationships*, Allyn & Bacon, Boston.

Heidegger, M. 1996, *Being and Time: A Translation of Sein und Zeit*, trans. J. Stambaugh, State University of New York Press, Albany.

Levinas, E. 1961, *Totality and Infinity: An Essay on Exteriority*, trans. A. Lingis, vol. 24, Duquesne Studies Philosophical Series, Duquesne University Press, Pittsburgh.

Nietzsche, F. 1973, *Beyond Good and Evil: Prelude to a Philosophy of the Future*, trans. R. J. Hollingdale, Penguin, Harmondsworth.

Rorty, R. 1979, *Philosophy and the Mirror of Nature*, Princeton University Press, New Jersey.

Stoter, D. J. 1998, 'Spirituality', in S. Hinchcliff, S. Norman, & J. Schober (eds), *Nursing Practice and Health Care: A Foundation Text*, 3rd edn, Arnold, London, pp. 274–90.

Waldfogel, S. 1997, 'Religion and spirituality in the primary care setting: Towards the 21st century', in L. Hoyle (ed.), *Biopsychosocial Approaches in Primary Care: State of the Art and Challenges for the 21st Century*, Plenum Press, New York, pp. 201–16.

4

Dying the Way We Live

Jenny Hockey

Enabling people to die in social contexts that do not alienate them from the relationships and belief systems that have sustained them in earlier life is an important principle of palliative care (Samarel 1995). A life-threatening illness can raise the prospect of coming adrift from the embodied self we previously recognised as 'me' (Holstein & Gubrium 2000). Giddens uses the term 'ontological insecurity' to describe this fear (1991), something we may experience at any point in the lifecourse, but are particularly vulnerable to as we face death. As a result our faith in a belief system or a core relationship may waver, while new questions of meaning become pressing. Lawton, for example, reports a loss of religious commitment among hospice patients who were unable to reconcile the suffering they experienced and witnessed with their faith (2000, p. 176). Sheldon (1997) notes that the beliefs that were important in earlier life can change, for example, after migration: fourth-generation Black British people may share the values of the White population (1997, pp. 17–18). If illness undermines a lifetime's confidence in the body and, for example, erodes the body's boundaries (Lawson 2000), then we may cease to feel continuity with the person we grew up to be. This loss is but an extreme version of more mundane risks to ontological security caused by breakdowns in our social competence at any point in the lifecourse. As Giddens argues, '[b]odily self-management ... has to be so complete and constant that all individuals are vulnerable to moments of stress when competence breaks down—and the framework of ontological security is threatened' (1991, p. 57).

Thus, although palliative care may seek to sustain the way we live during the process of dying, someone's changed situation may, in itself, reinforce, reawaken, *or* quench their spiritual values, their commitments, purposes, and meaning. The material in this chapter speaks to two interlinked questions. First, how can we help people to draw upon resources that sustained them in crises earlier in their lives? Second, are the resources of earlier life actually relevant or accessible to people undergoing the physiological, emotional, and social changes that dying can bring? To explore these issues this chapter foregrounds the experiences of people nearing the ends of their lives, using pseudonyms to protect the confidentiality of individuals and institutions. It differs from work which, although addressed to religious needs, remains uneasily aware of both the diversity and the absence of religious commitment among patients. At the same time, it also avoids retreating into highly individualistic accounts that emphasise the uniqueness of each patient's experience of the dying process but leave carers ill prepared.

Before considering how to escape these two pitfalls, we need to recognise the lack of any easy consensus as to what the concept of 'spiritual needs' actually means (Walter 1994, 1997; Bradshaw 1996). Indeed, we can ask why this particular thread from the fabric of a previous life should be unravelled for scrutiny. The dying process is often thought of as a period when hard spiritual questions about the meaning of life and the fate of the soul become urgent (Parkes 1997; Sheldon 1997). Yet this view assumes that questions made central by the world's faiths are hardwired into the human psyche, ready to surface whenever death becomes inevitable. This limited, functionalist definition of religion reduces it to a coping strategy for beings blessed or cursed with awareness of their own mortality. If palliative care wishes to sustain the way we live during the dying process, then even sidestepping religious frameworks to focus on broader questions about the meaning of life risks reproducing the core priorities of the world's faiths. The notion of ontological security more usefully takes us to ground we can work from. As Taylor argues, '[i]n order to have a sense of who we are, we have to have a notion of how we have become, and of where we are going' (cited in Giddens 1991, p. 54). This sense of who we are involves faith in ourselves as worthwhile, independent beings and confidence that the external world of objects, people, and relationships actually is the way we have come to believe it is. This approach returns us to the question of whether terminal illness reinforces, reawakens, or quenches spiritual values, but recasts it in terms of self-identity, so redirecting us to the moral and biographical resources through which the individual previously achieved ontological security.

RELATING 'THE INDIVIDUAL TO THE SOCIAL

If narrow definitions of religion or assumptions about the urgency of big questions are potentially problematic, what happens if each individual is approached on his or her own terms? Many authors stress the importance of sensitivity to the individual. Sheldon cites Julia Neuberger's concern with the 'individual mix', which constitutes someone's unique relationship with one of the major religious faiths (1997, p. 19). Gunaratnam (1997) similarly warns against the healthcare profession's tendency towards a fact-file approach to cultural differences which ignores *individual* differences. Potted inventories of the beliefs and practices of particular faiths run the risk of reification and the construction of 'one-dimensional snapshots of cultural and religious practices which are frozen in both time and context' (1997, p. 170). However, while stressing that professionals should instead respond to patients as individuals, Gunaratnam also makes what is a key point for the present volume—that dying is a social and therefore interpersonal process. As such it can involve relations of power and inequality. Thus those who die as they live sometimes find themselves in conflict with the interests of healthcare professionals and the patients who share the dying space of a hospital or hospice ward. For example, the nurses who took part in Gunaratnam's focus groups reported that both patients and staff found it 'difficult', 'frightening', 'demanding', and 'stressful' to witness large numbers of bereaved people conducting loud rituals of mourning, in an apparently 'raw' emotional state (1997, p. 181). In this example, conflicts turned on issues of race, but differences of class, gender, sexuality, and age can similarly bring unequal relations of power into play.

Gunaratnam's refusal of these two problematic positions—'culture as fact-file' and 'the individual as unique'—opens the way for a social and cultural analysis of what is said and done by particular patients, their families, and their carers. It overcomes the tension between two unsatisfactory approaches to spiritual care—the one reducing individual experience to a cultural stereotype, the other abstracting the individual from his or her *social* life. Interestingly, this tension is not restricted to practitioners but is one that social scientists have struggled with since the emergence of their disciplines at the turn of the twentieth century. The sociologist Emile Durkheim, for example, sought to differentiate his findings from philosophical or psychological accounts of human behaviour by identifying the social as something over and above the sum of society's individual members. However, more recent work has challenged accounts of society as an external force, which determines and defines individual behaviour, and called for explanations of how society's individual members actually *make* the society they inhabit. Of relevance for spiritual care is the recent anthropological collection *Questions of Consciousness* (Cohen & Rapport 1995), which argues that '[t]o pay attention to the consciousness of the individual and to the narratives in which it is expressed is *not* to privilege the individual over society, but, rather, is a necessary condition for the sensitive understanding of social relations and of society as composed of, and constituted by, subjective individuals in interaction' (1995:11–12). Like Gunaratnam (1997), therefore, these authors identify the social or interactive dimensions of inner thoughts and feelings.

This reconciliation between the individual and the social at the theoretical level clearly offers something to the practitioner faced with religious, spiritual, and cultural differences between individuals. It provides an alternative to fruitless debates which separate out and then privilege either culture or the individual and so risk misunderstanding both. Rapport shows us that behaviours that are highly specific to an individual can still be understood as part of something collective or social. He says that 'the collective structures of social *reality* can only be fully grasped through an appreciation of the way they are personalised in individual lives' (1993, p. 165). In other words, social forms—for example, the content of fact-files about different religious beliefs and practices—only come to life and acquire meaning as social reality when individuals take them up according to their own motivations and agendas. Rapport goes on to say that 'behavioural commonalities are personalised in usage and come to be animated in possibly idiosyncratic fashions. They become instruments of diversity and difference, and yet the conditions of their use remain essentially public' (Rapport 1993, p. 170).

It is this approach that the current chapter adopts. We begin with the findings from studies among different categories of people nearing the ends of their lives. These show that social differences—age, region, gender, and religious affiliation—can be broadly linked with particular kinds of cultural resources. However, we need to remember that social reality is produced by individuals drawing upon these cultural resources according to their own needs and agendas—an approach that meshes with the practical concerns of carers providing spiritual support for individuals. Starting at the broad level of cultural differences, we will then move on from these data to examine the way individuals animate their culture's repertoire of social forms.

This approach is paralleled in Gunaratnam's plea that Black and ethnic minority patients be recognised as 'active subjects whose subjective and materially influenced performances can reaffirm, modify and challenge cultural scripts' (1997, p. 179). It also meshes with a lifecourse approach that makes the intersection of collective history and individual biography its focus. With this conception of the social we gain a sense of the agency of individuals who not only make choices during the dying process but also get to exercise power in unanticipated or unrecognised ways.

Debates about spiritual care within the hospice literature often address the dilemmas of providers rather than users (Walter 1994,1997; Bradshaw 1996). They ask which staff should be responsible and whether spiritual care might become a focus for audit. Should it dovetail with nursing care or would it become either indistinguishable from empathic support or problematic for nurses who do not share patients' beliefs? If left to the chaplain, would it become more exclusive and less flexible (Walter 1994, 1997; Bradshaw 1996)? What the data included in this chapter remind us, however, is that patients themselves may determine not only what the spiritual is about, but also how making the spiritual visible might allow their personal agendas to be met.

CULTURAL REPERTOIRES

Studies of the social and cultural dimensions of death and dying among the members of different social categories and cultures differ in terms of respondents' closeness to death. Yet, as Kellehear notes, the criterion of 'dying' itself is not always easy to apply (1990, p. 66). People can live with a 'terminal illness' for up to thirty years. Kellehear himself chose social identity as his focus, interviewing people who thought of themselves as dying and felt they had 'an abnormally shortened sense of future time in which to live' (1990, p. 66).

Other studies have taken a more distanced position. We begin with Williams's account of attitudes to death and illness among older Aberdonians. Williams uses qualitative data from interviews with seventy people over the age of 60 to identify the 'moral and economic resources that Aberdonians turn to when they think about how to cope with physical limitation and loss—with illness, ageing, and death' (1990, p. 1). As such, the data are tied to a particular time and place and reveal an intertwining of older people's economic and religious histories, which together produce particular responses in the present. Crucially for this chapter, Williams stresses that his focus is 'not directly on coping but on conceptions of how to cope' (1990, p. 10). In other words, his data describe the repertoire of values and beliefs available to people—though not necessarily how they draw upon them when faced with life-threatening illnesses. What Williams identifies is the importance of a work ethic which, although varying across classes, predominated among a generation whose core experiences of employment took place in the years following the Second World War. Attitudes were further shaped by one of two traditions: 'either by a typically activist self-image or by ethical or religious convictions deriving mainly from the Protestant tradition' (1990, p. 316). Interviewees represented a population divided between Christians and nonbelievers and between different Christian views. This was reflected in a range of conceptions of how to approach death, comprising a Calvinist model of ritual dying after lifelong preparation, a more general preparedness for a natural death, a natural death which takes the individual unawares, and, finally, personal awareness and control over the dying process. What Williams stresses, however, is that in practice individuals would draw on— and draw together—apparently contradictory approaches.

During an anthropological study among forty-five very elderly people living in residential care in the northeast of England (Hockey 1989; 1990), I found a similar continuity of values across time. Using both participant observation and interviewing among people who had actually been admitted to institutional care, I could examine the way these values resourced residents' strategic management of present circumstances, for example, providing a code of conduct for surviving difficult times or helping explain how the lifecourse had culminated in particular forms of illness or deterioration. Like those in Williams's sample, most residents had not been diagnosed as dying, yet a quarter of them did die during the ten-month period of study, a not unusual death rate within this home. Living in institutional care, their relationship with death was closer than that among the Aberdonians.

In interviews residents made an explicit differentiation between 'then' and 'now', between their earlier, independent lives and their current institutional location. This provided the basis for their time-based interpretive framework, a resource through which they constructed not only a way of managing but also an explanation for their current difficulties. For example, I observed Ethel Carr, a single woman of 84, dealing with an unwelcome transition to old age and residential care by befriending selected residents who would not make too many demands on her. When interviewed, she stressed the importance of 'true friendship and true neighbourhood', values that she located in the past. 'Ah, but you know, people were different in them days to what they are now.' Ethel also explained her current loss of independence in terms of her hard life as a single woman running a bakery and confectionery business. She identified her strict mother as the reason she never had a family of her own: 'Mothers shape their daughters' destinies,' she asserted.

Arthur Grant, an 82-year-old former schoolteacher, Methodist, and veteran of the First World War, managed his waning physical health and the gradual loss of many members of his family through stoicism and independence. He described his strict upbringing, which strictness he had later reproduced as a disciplinarian schoolteacher. Though military service had undermined his health, it also provided a code for managing adversity: 'Just have to square up to it', 'I'm not grumbling', and 'I get through. I know what to do. You know yourself. You know what to do.' Just as Ethel asserted the values of true friendship and true neighbourhood in 'them days', so Arthur compared carol singing in the 1900s with the lost spirit of Christmas today. 'Pelting snow, didn't matter—we still went—great days! The spirit of Christmas was alive then—there *was* a spirit. There's not now, there's not now. No wonder we enjoyed it.' And, like Ethel, long-distant events helped explain current difficulties. When I asked him what he put his loss of mobility down to, he said, 'Just the wear and tear of war, I would say. Course there's thousands and thousands of miles we used to walk—march. No wonder. Course up in the Alps—we had two horrid winters, frostbitten right to the ankles, dead ... Two and a half years in Italy. Made a wreck of me. Came back with nothing—not a halfpenny—no money.' Generalising to other men of his generation in the institution, he said, 'It's very noticeable now that the three of us in here that were in the First [World] War—there's George, big Jimmy and meself—all our legs, they're going. Sometimes we can't walk. They're afflicted in the same way.'

Looking back from the perspective of the present, he said, 'Nobody would believe it, nobody would believe it. We're suffering for it now, but there we are ... Just have to square up to it, that's all. Frostbite. All for sixpence a day ... To think of the things that have happened—you wouldn't believe I'd charged across no man's land to kill a man. Kill or be killed!'

This stoicism was evident among the values of other residents. Sissy Crowther, a middle-class woman in her eighties who had been a voluntary worker, decorated for organising canteen services in the Second World War, described her despair at the prospect of gradual decline into physical dependency. She felt she had little to look forward to, but finished her conversation with me by asserting that she would just have to *make* herself happy. An age-based, generational identity was therefore asserted by these residents, earlier values being shown to hold their worth in present-day adversity, past events providing causal explanations for current ill health or loneliness.

These data show residents sharing strategies that allowed them to repair a damaged sense of ontological security through narratives of the past that made sense of present circumstances. Stoicism and independence, coupled with more vivid forms of sociality, were core to many recollections of 'them days'. However, gender also intersects with age within these data. While men drew on work histories and their involvement in local organisations such as the church or concert party groups, women identified themselves in terms of relationships that had sustained them—and actively grieved those of which they had been bereaved. Some men sustained their public identities in modified form—rehearsing the residents' choir, selling newspapers, growing plant cuttings for sale, and representing fellow residents on the institution's committee. For women whose lives had been domestically grounded, this role was felt to be usurped by domestic and care staff who ironed, made beds, and cooked, a gender-based difference that was also evident in Evers's study of women patients in long-stay geriatric wards (1981).

In work on gender, ageing, and spirituality, however, King (1999) argues that feminism has led women of all ages into a concern with holism and integration—in the form of the womanspirit movement or spiritual feminism. We can speculate that rather than dwelling on a sense of loss as domestic and family roles become untenable, spirituality will, for some women, continue to be an important resource at the ends of their lives. Komaromy's work among older people in residential care (Komaromy & Hockey 2001) reveals that in Quaker homes female residents may well be former Roman Catholics who changed their beliefs or, as one head of home put it, 'found their right religion before they died'.[1] This head of home stated that, 'They have a lot of ex-Catholics, the Friends do, especially women because, as you know, the Catholic church doesn't necessarily give them a very good deal, does it?'

Kellehear's study of social behaviour and experiences among a sample of 100 Australians who were dying of cancer provides data about a population for whom ' "dying" was part of their new and final social identity' (1990, p. 65). His findings revealed the importance of religious frameworks for people in this context. Rather than conceptions of how one should or might cope, these data derive from people who know they are living through the experience of dying.

Just as the Aberdonians' coping strategies were informed by a collective religious history traceable to the sixteenth century and the Reformation, so one-third of Kellehear's sample drew on their *personal* histories of religious involvement when faced with death, reviving lapsed practices of prayer, churchgoing and involvement with clergy.

By way of contrast, religious beliefs and practices were unimportant for the hospice patients among whom Lawton worked (2000). Her sample included people with particularly distressing bodily symptoms, for example, chronic diarrhoea and vomiting. It was this breakdown of the body's boundaries that secured them a place within a hospice facing heavy demand for its services. Another important aspect of their identity was their class background, of which Lawton says, 'Even after patients had lost many attributes of self due to their illness and deterioration, class appeared to be the one aspect of *themselves* which many retained more or less right up until the point of death' (2000, p. 35). Her material reveals the importance of bodily boundaries for self-identity, their loss threatening ontological security to the extent that a 'debasement and erosion of their personhood', 'a loss of self', took place. In these circumstances patients came adrift from the moral or biographical resources of earlier life, their changed bodily condition producing an unbearable contrast with the 'me' they had previously been. A woman whose breast cancer surgery meant the temporary exposure of her rib cage and heart said that even after skin grafts she could no longer bear to look at her 'mutilated body' (2000, p. 45). Lawton describes dying patients who refused food and any form of social contact, who became 'dead' to staff, family, and friends. Even core markers of social differentiation such as gender were undermined by bodies that no longer conformed to notions of femininity or masculinity, either in appearance or practice. Yet, class differences often remained, working-class patients preferring the company and the attention on shared wards, middle-class patients seeking the privacy of side rooms. However, Lawton suggests that this distinction was externally sustained by staff who used social class as an implicit criterion when allocating ward space.

Individual and social integration: a lifecourse approach

Harris describes the lifecourse as the coming together of individual biography and collective history, a 'total social process which has both collective and individual moments' (1987, p. 66). Almost ten years earlier Johnson had argued for an approach to human ageing that took account of 'the historical roots of personal "needs" ' (1978, p. 106). What concerned him was gerontology's tendency to homogenise older people on the basis of age, ignoring the past experiences and processes that constitute the individual's unique biography. His critique of a misleading emphasis on 'the commonality of certain characteristics and experiences' (1978, p. 106) echoes social scientists' concerns about the privileging of gender, ethnic identity, age, or illness status to the neglect of the individuals who animate or inhabit these broad categories. To meet the needs of older adults effectively, Johnson advocates listening to their reconstructed biographies and finding out how their present issues have been sculpted by the values and experiences that made up their lifecourse. Johnson has since developed the concept of 'biographical pain'. He prefers this to 'spiritual pain' since the latter can be a residual category or catchall for suffering that escapes the categories of physical and psychological pain (1999). The concept of biographical pain, however, usefully alerts carers to the anguish of intractable interpersonal tensions, residual guilt, and unresolved grief. Komaromy's work on the management of death in residential homes (Komaromy & Hockey 2001) shows how residents are sometimes involved in planning their own care. One head of home said, 'I mean, there are a number of residents here that have done their own care plans and they've done a life story because they are quite capable of writing down. There are others that are unable to—but we get past history if they are not able to tell us … from the relatives … because it has a bearing on their continuing care.'

As Rapport argues, social reality is produced by individuals in interaction, the animation of social forms according to the individual's 'goals, motives, purposes, interests' (1993, p. 164). Having profiled data that point up differences of age, gender, region, religious affiliation, and health status, we now move on to look more closely at the personal orientations of individuals facing death and the repertoires of beliefs and practices which they draw upon in pursuing them. As argued, debates about spiritual care often privilege the concerns of providers. Yet, as the following data show, individuals facing death not only offer clear pointers as to their own spiritual and existential concerns but also exercise considerable agency in so doing.

FACING DEATH

To be close to death is a social identity that can represent both a resource and a threat, depending upon the interpersonal context in which its proximity is addressed. In the northeast residential home (Hockey 1990), staff were ill prepared and unsupported when it came to responding to older people's feelings about death. Silenced as a topic, death nonetheless became a resource that residents would draw upon to exercise power in situations that they experienced as disempowering—being fed, bathed, walked up the corridors, tucked up in a bed with bars. By making asides about death at the end of conversations individuals could have the last word, thereby silencing and embarrassing care staff. They would tell staff to sweep them up too along with the food scraps under the diningroom tables, ask a care assistant to push them under in the bath, or silently cross their arms on their chests when early morning tea was brought in, so simulating the corpse they would soon become (Hockey 1990). What stands out from these data is the agency of people who are faced with the prospect of their own mortality.

In the minority of residential homes where death and dying is framed within the context of either religious or psychotherapeutic discourses, residents discover a different form of agency, one that is realised as part of a very different relationship with staff. For example, in a south of England Quaker home for elderly people, a head of home discussed a resident, Emily Hulme, who had always contributed to the running of the institution. When the head of home was bereaved of her second husband, Emily drew on her 'institutional' identity as a practical helper, her personal experience of losing *her* second husband, and a lifetime's Quaker practice. She sent for the head of home, saying:

> I feel led to say something to you which will probably upset you … You keep doing things, don't you, you keep going to work, you keep doing the washing up, you tidy up the cupboard again … you must take time each day even to just sit quietly and think of all the lovely times … although you will feel upset at first it will make you feel very comfortable in the end. I just feel I must leave it with you … I will pass that on …

In a small, private residential home in the south of England, where psychotherapeutic care was emphasised, the head of home described the spiritual message she had received from residents:

> I was getting sort of burn out and I realised what was happening … I mean I was getting totally exhausted, more than I ever had done before … I realised what was happening was that we had several … people who were fairly frail and that I was working harder and harder to try and keep them going and actually … they were giving me a message, saying that they didn't want to go on and I needed to sort of hear that.

One resident made her readiness to die apparent. The staff member said, 'I realised when I took her tea in to turn her that she was actually going to die and I rang her daughter locally and she came and we sat with her and she just went and it was very wonderful because she didn't really die of anything specific.' The head of home had previously talked to the resident about dying and reported that, 'She said she was ready, she wanted to go. She wasn't in pain or discomfort, just weary.'

In the data presented in this section, people who are facing death raise the issue of their own mortality within the context of particular relationships with carers. In some contexts they actually offer spiritual care to staff, rather than the reverse. Death's associations with waste, timeliness, release, and relief are among the cultural representations that individuals animate for particular reasons—for example, to empower themselves via the capacity to silence or support someone occupying a structurally stronger position. This chapter has provided a social and cultural analysis of spiritual care-giving which, while acknowledging cultural differences, gives priority to the way in which individuals themselves animate the particular cultures—and the repertoires of cultural forms—that they identify with. As such it challenges the notion of spiritual care as something which staff deliver, arguing instead that it is the product of social interaction, something that takes place within the flow of quite specific local agendas.

REFERENCES

Bradshaw, A. 1996, 'The spiritual dimension of hospice: The secularization of an ideal', *Social Science and Medicine*, vol. 43, no. 3, pp. 409–19.

Cohen, A. P. & Rapport, N. 1995, *Questions of Consciousness*, Routledge, London.

Evers, H. 1981, 'Care or custody? The experiences of women patients in long-stay geriatric wards', in B. Hutter & G. Williams (eds), *Controlling Women*, Croom Helm, London.

Giddens, A. 1991, *Modernity and Self-Identity*, Polity Press, Cambridge.

Gunaratnam, Y. 1997, 'Culture is not enough: A critique of multi-culturalism in palliative care', in D. Field, J. Hockey, & N. Small (eds), *Death Gender and Ethnicity*, Routledge, London.

Harris, C. 1987, 'The individual and society: A processual approach', in A. Bryman et al. (eds), *Rethinking the Life Cycle*, Macmillan, London.

Hockey, J. 1989, 'Residential care and the maintenance of social identity: Negotiating the transition to institutional life', in M. Jefferys (ed.), *Growing Old in the Twentieth Century*, Routledge, London.

—— 1990, *Experiences of Death: An Anthropological Account*, Edinburgh University Press, Edinburgh.

Holstein, J. & Gubrium, J. 2000, *The Self We Live By: Narrative Identity in a Postmodern World*, Oxford University Press, New York.

Johnson, M. 1978, 'That was your life: A biographical approach to later life', in V. Carver & P. Liddiard (eds), *An Ageing Population*, Hodder & Stoughton, in association with the Open University Press, Sevenoaks.

Johnson, M. 1999, 'Biographical pain at the end of life', unpublished paper presented at the 28th Annual Conference of the British Society of Gerontology, Bournemouth, 17–19 September.

Kellehear, A. 1990, *Dying of Cancer. The Final Year of Life*, Harwood Academic Publishers, Chur, Switzerland.

King, U. 1999, 'Spirituality, ageing and gender', in A. Jewell (ed.) *Spirituality and Ageing*, Jessica Kingsley, London.

Komaromy, C. & Hockey, J. 2001. ' "Naturalizing" death among older adults in residential care' in J. Hockey, J. Katz & N. Small (eds), *Grief, Mourning and Ritual*, Open University Press, Buckingham, pp. 73–81.

Lawton, J. 2000, *The Dying Process: Patients' Experiences of Palliative Care*, Routledge, London.

Parkes, C. M. 1997, 'Help for the dying and the bereaved', in C. M. Parkes, P. Laungani, & B. Young (eds), *Death and Bereavement Across Cultures*, Routledge, London.

Rapport, N. 1993, *Diverse World-Views in an English Village*, Edinburgh University Press, Edinburgh.

Samarel, N. 1995. 'The dying process', in H. Wass & R. A. Neimeyer (eds), *Dying: Facing the Facts*, Taylor & Francis, Washington, DC.

Sheldon, F. 1997, *Psychosocial Palliative Care: Good Practice in the Care of the Dying and Bereaved*, Stanley Thornes, Cheltenham.

Walter, T. 1994, *The Revival of Death*, Routledge, London.

—— 1997, 'The ideology and organization of spiritual care: Three approaches', *Palliative Medicine*, vol 11, pp. 21–30.

Williams, R. 1990, *A Protestant Legacy: Attitudes to Death and Illness Among Older Aberdonians*, Clarendon Press, Oxford.

NOTE

1   These data form part of a wider study: Siddell, M., Katz, J., & Komaromy, C. 1997, *Death and Dying in Nursing and Residential Homes for Older People: Examining the Case for Palliative Care*, unpublished Department of Health report.

5

Finding Life Through Facing Death

Douglas Ezzy

'Everyone's dying, darling.'

Rex, in Ezzy 2000, p. 613.

Illness narratives can take a variety of forms. There are contingent narratives that express people's beliefs about the origins of disease and illness and its implications for their lives, moral narratives that describe and help implement changes in their social identity resulting from illness, and core narratives that connect people's experiences with deeper cultural levels of meaning attached to suffering and illness (Bury 2001). An encounter with life-threatening illness will often—probably usually—catalyse narratives that span all three of these forms. These narratives, which prepare people to face death—to embrace or resist it—may also equip them to engage life in fresh ways, as is illustrated in this chapter from conversations with people living with HIV/AIDS (PLWHA).

I discuss here four types of illness narratives:

- restitution narratives
- chaos narratives
- Christian illness narratives
- New Age illness narratives.

The first three narrative types are linear illness narratives. They privilege a well-integrated story oriented towards certainty about the future. In contrast New Age illness narratives are polyphonic (literally 'many voiced'), that is, they accept that stories may be inconsistent and dissonant, oriented towards the present, and more comfortable with uncertainty about, and an inability to control, the future. This chapter is an extension of an earlier paper in which I first differentiated polyphonic illness narratives from linear illness narratives (Ezzy 2000).

Many contemporary studies of illness experience privilege a linear narrative structure, with a simple plot line oriented towards success in the future (Ezzy 2000). Linear illness narratives conceptualise illness as an interruption to be overcome so that normal life can be resumed. Illness is minimised, and the impact—or potential impact—of the illness is denied or discounted. Linear narratives tend to be secular, confident of the efficacy of medical science, and confident of the individual's ability to overcome. They can also be Christian; this is discussed in detail below. Hope in linear illness narratives refers to confidence in the future, preferably a long-term future. Death tends not to be discussed and, if it is discussed, it is conceptualised as a distant possibility. Linear illness narratives are well-told stories, they suppress contradiction and dissonance, and, through life review, provide a sense of satisfaction with a life well lived (Ezzy 1998). The main exemplar of a linear illness narrative here is the 'restitution' narrative.

A variation on the linear narrative is the 'chaos' narrative (Frank 1995), or narrative of loss (Crossley 1999). These illness stories retain the *ideal* of a linear narrative. Narrators want to be made well, to be able to minimise the effects of their illness, *but* the severity of their symptoms or the consequences of their diagnosis makes this impossible. Chaos narratives are stories of the failure of medical science to solve the problems that these people believe medical science should be able to solve. In chaos narratives death, and the anticipation of death, is an indicator of failure.

Christian illness narratives are a third variant of the linear illness narrative. Secular linear illness narratives colonise the future through a confidence in medical science and the heroic strength of the individual. Christian illness narratives colonise the future through faith in an afterlife and the religious actions of the individual. Weber (1976) argued some time ago that there was an elective affinity between protestant Christianity and the secular spirit of capitalism. The linear narrative structure shared by Christian, restitution, and chaotic illness narratives reflects this affinity.

In contrast, polyphonic narratives are characterised by 'overlaid, interwoven and often contradictory stories and values' (Ezzy 2000, p. 613). These narratives interweave the pain of loss with the joy of new discoveries, and the pleasure of surprise and shared happiness. There is a recognition that not everything is under the control of human agents and an acceptance of the limited nature of medical science. Hope is not associated with the distant future, but with the celebration of surprise and mystery in the present. Davies (1997) refers to this as 'living with a philosophy of the present'. Polyphonic narrators accept the inevitability of mortality and are comfortable with the idea that they may die soon. The main exemplar of a polyphonic illness narrative discussed here is the New Age illness narrative.

It is common to distinguish spirituality—universally shared and referring to the central domains of human values and meaning—from religion—systems of belief and practice that ritualise and institutionalise spirituality (Mount 1993). This definition of spirituality is, however, rather vague. In order to analyse the spiritual dimensions of illness narratives, Kellehear's (2000) three types of spiritual needs relevant to palliative care are useful: situational, moral/biographical, and religious. Situational needs include the need to give the illness experience meaning and to provide a sense of hope that transcends the current situation; this may also be related to social needs. Moral and biographical needs include the desire to set right past wrongs, to reconcile estranged companions, and to provide a sense of integration to one's life as a part of life review. Religious needs refer to the overt practices and beliefs of past and current religious practice that may require appropriate rituals or discussion. Kellehear suggests that different people will seek to address different spiritual needs through a process of transcendence. How four types of illness narratives provide—or do not provide—spiritual transcendence in these three categories of spiritual need identified by Kellehear will be demonstrated in this chapter.

RESEARCHING NARRATIVES

The four illness narrative types were identified as part of an ongoing qualitative study of living with HIV/AIDS in Australia funded by a National Health and Medical Council Research Grant (GN 990621). The interviews reported here were conducted between 1997 and early 2000 and included forty indepth interviews of PLWHA from Melbourne, Sydney, and Tasmania, some of whom were interviewed two or three times over the study period. Interviewees were asked a series of questions about employment history, illness experience, religious beliefs, and their understanding of the future. The indepth interviews were typically an hour in duration, were taped, transcribed, and analysed using grounded theory (Orona 1990) and narrative theory (Rice & Ezzy 1999).

There is a wide variety of definitions of what constitutes a narrative and an equally wide variety of approaches to the analysis of these narratives (Riessman 1993). Here, the term 'narrative' refers to the metaphorical construction of a story about past, present, and future; this narrative is built up throughout the interview. The method of analysis followed that employed by Frank (1995), focusing on the shape or form of the narrative as a whole. The narrative analysis involved identifying the dominant narrative structure around which each interview was formed. The typology of narrative forms presented below was developed inductively through detailed reflection on the characteristics of each narrative, comparison of the narratives, and, finally, grouping them into similar types based on shared temporal orientations and plot structure.

SPIRITUALITY, TIME, AND HIV/AIDS

A national survey of PLWHA in Australia in 1997 found that they often reported developing spiritual beliefs as a consequence of their diagnosis (Ezzy 2000). This is consistent with other studies of spirituality and illness. Taylor et al. (1995, p. 39), for example, summarise their literature review observing that 'people with cancer often report an increased sense of spirituality, a rise in existential concerns, and a use of religion as a coping strategy'. The national survey of PLWHA also found that, independent of indicators of disease progression, spiritual belief was associated with the extent of future planning. Specifically—and surprisingly—spiritual belief was associated with short-term planning (Ezzy 2000).

Spiritual belief among PLWHA splits roughly three ways, with slightly more than a third identifying themselves as atheists and agnostics (39 per cent), a third Christians (36 per cent), and slightly less than a third identified with New Age or New Age-like beliefs (25 per cent) (for example, Buddhist, Pagan, Sufi, spiritual). Consistent with the findings of other studies of New Age beliefs (York 1995), Buddhist PLWHA are considered a variant of New Age-like beliefs because typically they did not have a family history of Buddhism and were not connected to a Buddhist congregation. The link between Buddhism and the New Age is also consistent with the influence of Buddhist thought on New Age approaches to death (Walter 1993).

In summary, the national survey of PLWHA identified that spirituality is an important part of many people's response to a diagnosis. Second, spiritual belief is often associated with short-term planning. This suggests that spiritual beliefs facilitate the temporal reframing of life narratives. More specifically, it suggests that spiritual beliefs are associated with an acceptance of mortality. These points will be examined in detail in the remainder of this chapter, including how four types of illness narrative are associated with different understandings of death and the future and facilitate—or fail to facilitate—three types of spiritual transcendence identified by Kellehear (2000): situational, moral/biographical, and religious.

Disease progression among PLWHA is indicated by both viral load (if this is below 10 000, the rate of disease progression is slow) and T-cell counts (if this is below 200, HIV has done considerable—possibly irreversible—damage to the immune system).

RESTITUTION NARRATIVES

I interviewed Bill twice, once in 1997 and once in 1999. Bill is a gay man who was 38 years old at the first interview and had been infected and diagnosed for two years. His serological indicators were excellent (at both interviews he reported T-cells of 800 and an undetectable viral load). He was confident that he would live to an old age and that medical developments would ensure that HIV did not shorten his life. This attitude was clearest in his response to questions about how he thought about the future. He explicitly denied that HIV had shaped his understanding of the future. The complexity of his reflections on the other factors that have influenced his feelings about the future suggest that this is not simply a denial of the impact of HIV on his life, but a reflection of his genuine confidence in the efficacy of medical treatment. Whether this confidence is justified is difficult to evaluate.

> *I*　You said your understanding of the future has changed. Why do you think that is?
>
> *B*　I don't know that it's AIDS related, if you know what I mean. I think I'm feeling really comfortable about being 40, going into the next 10 years. Old age still scares me though … I'm really happy with how I'm looking physically with … like, I feel more settled in my career options … I can be quite comfortable on the money I make. The house is slowly getting finished and paid off, so I've got a roof over my head. If all else fell to bits I'd be OK and I think that's made me feel very comfortable and very sure

of myself. I haven't resolved the thing about do I want a partner in my life ... maybe it's friends that I want to have around in old age, not necessarily a lover ... I think I feel quite confident about the HIV as well. I think there's a definite future there. And growing old is not quite as fearful as it was 10 years earlier.

Bill's story about the future revolves around assumptions of normal ageing and the influence of his work, home ownership, and relationships. HIV enters as an afterthought. The goals that he describes are continuations of goals developed prior to his diagnosis. That is to say, his life is normalised as much as possible to be consistent with the life expectations of people without HIV/AIDS.

Bill's narrative also emphasises his confidence in the efficacy of the treatments available to people with HIV/AIDS. In 1996 a new set of treatments for HIV/AIDS became available; they are referred to as combination therapy, or simply 'the new treatments'. Bill's confidence in these treatments may reflect the opinion of some doctors who are equally hopeful that the new treatments will turn HIV into a manageable chronic illness. While these treatments have improved many PLWHAs' health, and death rates have significantly declined, their long-term efficacy is frustratingly uncertain (Flexner 1998).

Bill's narrative is a strong version of the restitution narrative. Weaker versions of the restitution narrative are more accepting of a limited lifespan and set goals commensurate with this. While the strong version of the restitution narrative typically tries to avoid a consideration of mortality, as a person comes to accept the possibility of death, it can lead to a secular acceptance of mortality, although restitution narratives typically retain a focus on goals to be achieved in the future. Other participants hoped, for example, to live long enough to see their children leave home, or to finish a course of study, or to achieve some other normal goal.

Restitution narratives provide a sense of situational transcendence through reinstating or reclaiming normal life goals as achievable, despite the illness or uncertain prognosis. While life may be partially integrated through life review, the temporal focus of restitution narratives is firmly on the anticipated, and colonised, future. Restitution narratives link a satisfying life to the achievement of these future goals. Consistent with the enlightenment narrative of modernist science, death, if it is contemplated, is reduced 'from the basic religious problem of the human being, to a series of discrete—and hopefully curable—medical conditions' (Walter 1993, p. 128). Within the framework of the restitution narrative, religious transcendence through rituals or traditional beliefs tends to be discounted as irrelevant.

At the heart of restitution narratives lies an uncomfortable tension between the desire for a socially sanctioned 'normal' life and the uncertainty of prognosis. This tension is not simply a personal trouble, but also a public issue, born of contemporary society's obsession with colonisation of the future (Giddens 1991). This tension was poignantly underlined later in the interview when Bill mentioned, as an aside, that there were some aspects of HIV that still scared him.

> *I* You said you were scared. What do you mean?
>
> *B* I was really surprised when that [the word 'scared'] popped into my mind. Maybe vulnerable would be a better word. Although I'm quite confident, there's still some niggling doubts. There's still that fear of what happens if … the what ifs, you know. And not only for me, but I'm quite scared for some of my friends. This year I've been to four funerals. I've been seeing people who are failing [on the treatments] where they shouldn't … So I think that's shaken me up just a little bit to have these number of deaths. We've got this total reliance that these pills will save us, but maybe they won't.

Bill underlines that treatment failure should not be happening, and that confidence about his life and his future is integrally bound up with an almost overconfident trust in medical technology.

CHAOS NARRATIVES

Lex is a 47-year-old manual labourer who was infected seventeen years ago. Although his seriological indicators were excellent (an undetectable viral load and T-cells of 700), he was struggling with depression, in part as a consequence of the deaths of most of his network of friends.

> *L* I had known a lot of people who were acquaintances and friends of friends or some friend's lover in what you call my [gay] family, who'd gotten ill and died. The last Mardi Gras party I went to was with Graham. He looked dreadful. He was on AZT and high doses back then and really deteriorating, but he wanted to be at the party so we went. But, other people kept coming up to me and saying, 'I didn't know Graham was so

ill', because they hadn't seen him. So I pretty much kept to my group of friends since then. I don't go out as much. So, I'm pretty depressed about it. And getting more depressed about it, I think. Like, it was such a heavy downer. I think I've become numb. I was coping by ignoring it, too ... The important thing is spending time with friends and lovers. That ... that was the big thing of being gay and openly gay. It's so important and having a family and people I loved for the first time. When they started dying, that was what was important. But then you've got to have a break from it. Sometimes you wouldn't go out because you might see someone.

I You said you get depressed?

L Well, I was clinically depressed. It was diagnosed by the doctor and I was on medications. It was only going to be about 3 or 4 months but I actually came off antidepressants after 6 years or so. Actually, I think I'll go back on them, because I don't think my depression is completely dissipated. I've always been an insomniac, so sleep has always been difficult. I'd have excessive mood swings, mainly in the negative. I become extremely self-critical and dwell on negative aspects of my life and situations. I have the physical effects of lethargy and a lack of desire to do anything.

I So how far into the future do you think?

L I don't make plans. I don't make plans at all. I've got my Mardi Gras ticket, but that's only because they sell ahead. If you don't buy them you won't get in.

Lex's chaos narrative is a narrative of loss and failure. His depression is a product of his inability to attain, in his real life, the story of a life of gay liberation, which he retains as an ideal. His ideal narrative is linear in the sense that Lex has a simple, clear story of progressive liberation. He contrasts his current life with this ideal and finds his current life to be a failure. Lex has lost a life as a gay man within a broader gay family that he found liberating and rewarding. This loss is not only the product of his illness, but also a product of the death of many of his friends. The specific content of the idealised linear life is culturally variable. Lex's ideal narrative revolves around parties and participation in the gay family. Heterosexual males often idealise success in their career and having a family. Similarly, for some women, the desire to have children is the focus of their idealised normal life, and career success is peripheral. Whether the ideal normal life involves a career and family, or parties and participation in gay culture, or having children, the pain—and chaos—of these narratives is a product of the collapse of normalised and desired lifeplans.

Chaos narratives focus on the failure of both situational and moral/biographical factors. In terms of situational needs, the understanding of the future is typically one of narrowing options and loss. Individuals report feeling socially isolated and stigmatised by their illness or association with the illness. In terms of moral and biographical needs, people often feel estranged from previously important communities and friends. One of the central issues for chaotic narrators is the difficulty of integrating their self-understanding around a lifeplan when their illness has destroyed—or threatens to destroy—the things that were central to their previous life narrative.

Both restitution narratives and chaos narratives rarely include any reference to religious beliefs or practice. When asked if they had any religious beliefs, people with chaotic narratives typically replied with an emphatic 'No'. Their response implied that it was almost ludicrous to suggest that religious belief might have a place in their self-understanding.

Serious illness, and associated bodily degeneration, confronts and ruptures a person's sense of independence, autonomy, and control. It breaks up the taken-for-granted experience of the world previously known through a healthy body, and disrupts the security systems against anxiety that assumed immortality (Mount 1993). Chaos narratives describe this disruption and provide no hope of resolution outside of the explicitly acknowledged vain hope of the restoration of a pre-illness life.

CHRISTIAN ILLNESS NARRATIVES

Allen is a 40-year-old gay man who was diagnosed in the late 1980s. His seriological indicators were good (viral load of 3000, T-cells of 500). He had been talking about his experience of the new treatments when he said:

> I don't know what's in store … But, having seen what I've seen and watched the people die that I have, I'm not frightened of it any more … Everyone's faced with death … the focus should be on life … I've always sort of liked to have thought that there's life after death, that life goes on, but I actually know that it does, I don't just believe it, I know it for a fact, so that's very comforting.

Allen then told the story of visiting a dying friend, Greg, who was also a close friend of his now deceased partner Terry. As Allen was leaving, Greg asked him, 'Allen? Do you want me to take a message to Terry for you? Is there anything you want me to tell him?' Allen said:

And I just looked at him—that just blew me away … There's this poor little sick, tiny little person who's dying in a bed, asking me if there was anything they could do for me … I was speechless for a while and I just thought I can't believe he's asking me this and I said to him, 'Well, no, not really, nothing special', I said, 'just tell Terry that I … you know … I miss him and that I still really love him.' And Greg, he just turned his head around to me and he said, 'Anything else?' He had a really strong accent, he was Maltese, and he said, 'Oh, Allen, don't you know that Terry knows that, he knows that already, and he's here?' And just as he said, 'He's here', Terry was there in the room and I knew exactly in the room where Terry was. I couldn't see him, I didn't have a vision or anything, but he was there and I could … I could even point where he was; he was standing, like, right by the door. And I knew he was there. I could feel him. All the hair on the back of my neck stood up. I just … it was fantastic. It was amazing. And I knew he was there and I knew he was okay … So I know life goes on. So that's death.

I asked Allen if he had any religious beliefs.

I'm a Christian, but I'm strictly non-denominational. My whole philosophy on religion is the story of the Good Samaritan. If you see someone who's in trouble and who's in need then you help them if you can. And that's what Christianity is about … Christianity's all about love, it's all based on love, forgiveness and kindness … instead we're all striving to accumulate our own private little wealth, have more than anyone else … the whole world's motivated by greed.

A little later in the interview Allen engaged in a form of life review in response to a question about how he understood his self-identity. I asked him to give me five or so words in response to the question 'Who am I?'

Opinionated [pauses five seconds]. Always right, of course [pauses eight seconds]. This is hard [pauses three seconds]. I'd like to think of myself as a considerate sort of person … I hope that I'm regarded as a good leader, of Positive People in this region, helping to empower them, helping to bring them to the negotiating table with the other stakeholders in the AIDS organisations … I hope I've been a good son [laughs].

Other participants typically provide either a list of roles, such as 'gay man', 'person living with HIV', or a list of personality characteristics, such as 'generous', 'caring', and so on. Allen begins this way, but then tells a story about his past and present that integrates them into a story that affirms the value of his life up to the present. The shift between present and past tense in the phrase 'I hope I've been a good son', is also indicative of the sense of closure provided by Allen's self-story. Rumbold (1989) points out that many people are able to come to terms with approaching death through a form of life review in which they tell a story about their life that constructs it as basically satisfying. Allen's narrative is just such an account.

Biographical integration reaches back into the past and into the future (Ezzy 1998). Knowing where you are going when you die meets the present need of being able to tell a story about your past life and your anticipated future. This story underlies both the value of the past life and the anticipated pleasure of what lies beyond the present. Christian illness narratives relinquish the need to plan for the future in this life, because they anticipate a future in the next life. It is therefore not surprising that Christian belief is associated with short-term planning.

Despite the correlation with short-term planning, Christian narratives still colonise the future in a similar way to the restitution narrative. The restitution narrative colonise the future through a faith in medical science and the efficacy of individual action. Christian illness narratives colonise the future through a faith in an afterlife and a confidence that the individual's faith will ensure entry to paradise. This faith, or religious transcendence, is a product of religious experience and/or ritual.

NEW AGE ILLNESS NARRATIVES

Rob is a 47-year-old gay man, diagnosed with HIV ten years before the interview. His seriological indicators were mixed (T-cells of 260, undetectable viral load).

I Are you religious?

R Spiritual would be more like it. I don't have any kind of religion, but if I had to embrace a religion it would be Zen Buddhism. It's a gentle religion, it's a practical religion. It's a religion of compassion. It's a way of being and this is what I found out of course when I was HIV positive is there is a certain amount of enlightenment goes on ... spiritually ... You question why you're here, for a start. You become more aware of other people's misfortune and so you become more in simpatico with your fellows ... You also become more confident. I'll sometimes talk at [public gatherings], which, I mean, normally I just wouldn't do something like that … It's a product of having a life-threatening illness. It's like these people who, you know, get cancer and suddenly find religion … I live more for the present [laughs].

New Age illness narratives describe a new spirituality that is intermingled with a changed understanding of time and a more compassionate attitude towards the suffering of others. Consistent with Davies's (1997) category of people who 'live with a philosophy of the present', New Age illness narratives celebrate the present. Levine's (1988) Buddhist-influenced New Age text on dying suggests that 'the aim—for the dying as for anyone—is to live in the present, attend to the present, accepting that everything changes' (Walter 1993, p. 136). Rather than striving to control the future, New Age illness narratives celebrate a transcendent hope in the surprise and pleasure of the present.

However, Rob recognised that HIV was not all wonderful. He particularly felt the difficulty of being poor and the difficulty of not being able to find a loving companion.

R I'm resigning myself to the fact that I may never ever have another lover. That I may never cohabitate with another man again. It's a very strange feeling. It's a sad feeling.

I Is there two sides to your story then?

R Yeah. It's been a good thing and it's been a bad thing. It's balanced out … HIV has been supremely important to myself as a human being. Very important to my emotional growth if you want a better phrase because some people … I mean, I found out this by experience … there's a lot of people out there who are emotionally bankrupt, you know, and who live life as a habit.

The complexity of the New Age illness narrative is important. It does not reduce the individual to a tragic pawn in the face of forces beyond any control, as does the chaos narrative. However, neither does it celebrate the agency of the individual through an attempt to control and colonise the future, as does the restitution narrative. As Levine (1988, p. 9) puts it, some 'events are, in a very real way, beyond our control'. In contrast to the linear nature of the other three narratives, New Age illness narratives tend to be polyphonic, with a greater sensitivity to the forces beyond human control that shape life.

Kennedy (1999), reflecting on Conigrave's (1995) autobiographical account of living with HIV/AIDS, points out that Conigrave's narrative is often disjointed, aesthetically awkward, and unsure of the overall central story. Kennedy (1999, p. 8) argues that these features of his narrative reflect Conigrave's own experience of the world 'as a disjointed set of characters, where he was unsure of how the parts of his life interconnected'. New Age illness narratives are typically, though not always, polyphonic (Ezzy 2000). They do not attempt to reconcile everything into a coherent story, preferring complexity, inconsistency, and ambiguity to the elision of integration.

The biographical—and moral—transcendence attained by New Age illness narratives is typically quite different in form to the transcendence of the linear narratives. Temporally, they celebrate the present rather than the future. People are seen as both agents able to influence their future and as at the mercy of forces beyond their control. Inconsistency and ambiguity are celebrated rather than avoided. Similar to the Greek tragic poets discussed by Nussbaum (1986), these narrators recognise values and definitions of the 'good' as plural and sometimes incommensurable. HIV/AIDS may have brought new spiritual insight, but this does not make the associated losses any less painful and difficult.

The religious transcendence of Christian illness narratives provides a personal rationale for the acceptance of a publicly shared religious belief system. The 'religious' transcendence of New Age illness narratives is more individualistic. Even the Buddhist spirituality that Rob draws upon is not grounded in a detailed knowledge of, or participation in, a religious institution with publicly shared beliefs. Hanegraaff (1999) suggests that New Age spirituality can be thought of as spirituality without religion for precisely this reason. However, New Age illness narratives do describe a form of religious transcendence through participation in a shared set of New Age beliefs that emphasise self-development and the rejection of the dualism of enlightenment modernism. Contrary to the pessimism of Hanegraaff, d'Epinay (1991) argues that the secular individualism that informs the emphasis on self-development of New Age spirituality can provide a robust foundation for ethics and justice.

New Age illness narratives typically included a criticism of the selfish materialism of both earlier periods in the narrator's life and of friends' lives. If the narrator's life was influenced *by* other people, concomitantly, the actions of the narrator had an important impact *on* other people. In contrast, the restitution and chaos narratives were typically oriented towards self-gratification and rarely described participation in political or community action. This is consistent with the emphasis of linear narratives on individual agency. In other words, it is not the New Age emphasis on 'nurturing the self' (York 1995) that leads to the decline of shared morality, rather, it is the linear modernist celebration of the rational autonomy of the subject that undermines shared values and political commitment.

Some commentaries on the place of New Age spirituality in palliative care appear to misunderstand the nature of the answers that New Age spirituality provides to the moral, biographical, and religious needs generated by illness and the anticipation of an early death. There is a tendency to assume that a religious response must take the form, if not the content, of one of the established religious traditions. For example, Walter (1993) assumes a modernist understanding of religion when he argues that New Age spirituality does not have the shared and socially given nature of other forms of spirituality and, as a consequence, does not provide the individual with a robust framework of meaning within which death can be interpreted. Walter (1993) and Hanegraaff (1999), are correct to point to the more pluralistic and fragile nature of New Age spirituality. However, this description of difference in form should not be read as a justification for professional prescription. The more uncertain, individualistic, and malleable nature of New Age spirituality does not make it a less worthwhile spiritual framework within which to make sense of one's life—and death. Rather, New Age spirituality would be better understood as a different cultural form to be valued in its own right.

CONCLUSION

Chaos illness narratives do not provide moral or autobiographical transcendence. As a consequence the chaotic narrators experience considerable spiritual anguish. The other narratives are all different resolutions to the shared spiritual need for situational, moral, and autobiographical transcendence. Restitution narratives provide moral and autobiographical transcendence through reinstating normalised life goals, with a focus on individual achievements in the future. Christian illness narratives find transcendence in a biographical integration that combines life review with a confidence in an afterlife. New Age illness narratives find transcendence in celebrating the present and in nurturing the self while questioning contemporary selfish materialism. It is important to note that the characteristics of Christian and New Age illness narratives, while representative of participants in my small sample, may be different among other groups. It is the properties of the narratives, rather than the particular religious traditions, that distinguishes them. It is quite possible to envisage Christian narratives that focus on the present, self-development, polyphony, and uncertainty, or New Age narratives that are dogmatic, modernist, and linear.

While traditional religious beliefs may be an important part of a person's illness narrative, they are not necessarily so. Such an insight is the product of applying a respect for complexity and uncertainty reflexively to our own practice. Mount (1993, p. 33) puts it well when he suggests that being part of the healing process involves developing 'a personal philosophy that can respect their right to be different … the most and the least we can do is to accompany them on their journey.' People are continually constructing and reconstructing the narratives within which they make sense of their lives. Care-givers often have the opportunity to participate in this process. Perhaps one of the most valuable contributions that can be made is simply to encourage people to tell a story without judging the content of that story. Even chaos narratives need to be heard, to be spoken, to allow the person who tells the story to express their pain.

Despair comes not simply from the failure to bring a life story to a potential close, but from the ontological disturbance to the narrative framing of a life that the acceptance of impending death brings. Spiritual illness narratives normalise death in a way that secular narratives find more difficult. Evidence for this comes from both the qualitative analysis of illness narratives and from the quantitative survey (Ezzy 2000) in which religious belief is associated with short-term planning, suggesting that religious belief facilitates the acceptance of the finite nature of a human life, at least in this world.

Hearing these stories—as care-giver or as researcher—elicits further narratives, illustrated by the following poem.

A Welcome Stranger

I sat quiet in the comfy chair,
'Twas near to dusk and before twilight.
Soft stillness hung in the air,
A glass of red calmed, anticipating the night.

A knock at the door broke my reverie,
Slowly my aging bones moved to welcome.
So little time left, yet so close to eternity,
I wondered at the intrusion into my home.

There she stood, eyes burning black, hair of red.
A shapely form, reeking of something unsettling me.

Agog at her beauty, yet terrified half dead.
I struggled to greet her with a modicum of decency.

'Why hello,' she flashed her smile and tossed her hair.
'Do come in,' I welcomed, feeling much more.
'Thank you,' she beamed, drawing my eyes to her chair.
I sat down too, no one shut the door.

As night closed and the crickets sang,
My seduced soul ebbed from terror to desire.
And in the heavily scented air, a funeral bell rang.
Almost calm, I knew what she would require.

'I am ready,' I said, meeting her gaze.
'Are you?' she queried, and raised an eyebrow.
So sensuous, my heart began churning, my mind a daze.
'Lead me gently, I'm sure you know how.'

We embraced and my eyes filled with tears.
The scent of her body and warmth of her skin,
Evoked lush memories from life's long years.
As my beating heart slowed she whispered: 'Shall we begin?'

'Hail and farewell,' I bade this life.
She opened a door with a black handled knife.
And as I stepped through and passed away.
I wondered, will you meet death in the same way?

Doug Ezzy

This poem is my response to interviewing, reading, and immersing myself in stories about living and dying with HIV/AIDS. Specifically, it was inspired by Marcus O'Donnell's (2000) obituary for Bill Phillips published in the *Sydney Star Observer*. O'Donnell reflects on the deep pain of Bill's dying, placing this pain beside Bill's poem 'The Angel of Death', which passionately describes the joy he anticipated in passing on. Similar to the story from *The Tales of the Arabian Nights*, my poem expresses something of what I have heard in the stories and lives of the people I interviewed: 'Sheherezade lives not by fighting the king or resigning herself to her fate but by engaging the heart and mind of that which might kill her' (Kellehear 2000, p. xviii). I have learnt to hear both the pain and the pleasure in the experiences of others as they face life-threatening illness; through their narratives their experiences become part of, and resonate with, my story. I too am encouraged to find life in facing death.

Healing, according to Mount (1993, p. 35), 'be it for the patient, family member or care-giver, may be defined as a process involving integration and transcendence, a process that enables expression of the unique essence at the core of personhood, and entry into dialogue'. This chapter has identified at least three ways of finding life through facing death, each with significantly different assumptions, beliefs, and temporal framing. As we talk and listen, we will discover a multitude of others.

> 'Hail and farewell,' I bade this life.
> She opened a door with a black handled knife.
> And as I stepped through and passed away.
> I was reminded, no one meets death in the same way.

REFERENCES

Bury, M. 2001, 'Illness narratives: Fact or fiction?', *Sociology of Health and Illness*, vol. 23, no. 3, pp. 263–85,

Conigrave, T. 1995, *Holding the Man*, McPhee Gribble, Melbourne.

Crossley, M. 1999, 'Stories of illness and trauma survival', *Social Science and Medicine*, vol. 48, no. 11, pp. 1685–95.

Davies, M. 1997, 'Shattered assumptions: Time and the experience of long-term HIV positivity', *Social Science and Medicine*, vol. 44, no. 4, pp. 561–71.

d'Epinay, L. 1991, 'Individualism and solidarity today: Twelve theses', *Theory, Culture and Society*, vol. 8, no. 1, pp. 57–74.

Ezzy, D. 1998, 'Lived experience and interpretation in narrative theory: Experiences of living with HIV/AIDS', *Qualitative Sociology*, vol. 21, no. 2, pp. 169–80.

—— 2000, 'Illness narratives: Time, hope and HIV', *Social Science and Medicine*, vol. 50, no. 5, pp. 605–17.

Flexner, C. 1998, 'HIV-protease inhibitors', *New England Journal of Medicine*, vol. 338, no. 9, pp. 1281–95.

Frank, A. 1995, *The Wounded Storyteller*, University of Chicago Press, Chicago.

Giddens, A. 1991, *Modernity and Self-Identity*, Stanford University Press, Stanford.

Hanegraaff, W. 1999, 'New Age spiritualities as secular religion', *Social Compass*, vol. 46, no. 2, pp. 145–60.

Kellehear, A. 2000, 'Spirituality and palliative care: A model of needs', *Palliative Medicine*, vol. 14, no. 1, pp. 149–55.

—— 2000, *Eternity and Me: The Everlasting Things in Life and Death*, Hill of Content, Melbourne.

Kennedy, S. 1999, 'Life review and heroic narrative: Embracing pathology and attention to context', *Australian and New Zealand Journal of Family Therapy*, vol. 20, no. 1, pp. 1–10.

Levine, S. 1988, *Who Dies?*, Gateway, Bath.

Mount, B. 1993, 'Whole person care: Beyond psychosocial and physical needs', *American Journal of Hospice and Palliative Care*, vol. 10, no. 2, pp. 28–37.

Nussbaum, M. 1986, *The Fragility of Goodness*, Cambridge University Press, Cambridge.

O'Donnell, M. 2000, 'Bill Phillips 1955–2000', *Sydney Star Observer*, 4 May, p. 13.

Orona, C. 1990, 'Temporality and identity loss due to Alzheimer's disease', *Social Science and Medicine*, vol. 30, no. 11, pp. 1247–56.

Rice, P. & Ezzy, D. 1999, *Qualitative Research Methods: A Health Focus*, Oxford University Press, Melbourne.

Riessman, C. 1993, *Narrative Analysis*, Sage, Newbury Park, California.

Rumbold, B. 1989, 'Spiritual dimensions in palliative care' in P. Hodder & A. Turley (eds), *The Creative Option of Palliative Care*, Melbourne Citymission, Melbourne, pp. 110–27.

Taylor, E., Amenta, M., & Highfield, M. 1995, 'Spiritual care practices of oncology', *Oncology Nursing Forum*, vol. 22, no. 1, pp. 31–9.

Walter, T. 1993, 'Death in the new age', *Religion*, vol. 23, no. 1, pp. 127–45.

Weber, M. 1976, *The Protestant Ethic and the Spirit of Capitalism*, trans. T. Parsons, George Allen & Unwin, London.

York, M. 1995, *The Emerging Network: A Sociology of the New Age and Neo-Pagan Movements*, Rowmann & Littlefield, Maryland.

Part 2

Reflecting upon Experience

Introduction

The relational basis of spirituality is here demonstrated in a series of personal accounts. Part 2 begins with chapter 6, an illness narrative placed in the context of a life story. In it, Maggie May recounts her experience of living with melanoma, showing how her encounter with a life-threatening illness is absorbed into—and contributes to the shaping of—her life and her vocation as an artist. Like the narratives of the participants in Ezzy's study (chapter 5), this account describes how living with life-threatening illness shapes perception and vocation. Such narratives clearly are not narratives in the last days of life, but the resources developed through this sort of reflection will profoundly influence those last days. To understand the diverse spiritual responses of people in palliative care programs we need to understand how these responses have developed in the encounter with life-threatening illness and how they express people's sense of their place in the world.

Chapters 7 and 8 present experiences of care-givers. Regina Millard (chapter 7) reflects on her role as a pastoral care worker in a palliative care program in Melbourne and the ways in which this has shaped her vocation and understanding of spirituality. Her account gives insight into the perspective, practice, and preparation of a pastoral care worker—helpful both for those who practise this discipline and those who work alongside pastoral care practitioners. She also chooses to speak about soul as the focus of spiritual care, a concept already alluded to in chapter 3 and developed in detail in Cobb's recent book, *The Dying Soul: Spiritual Care at the End of Life* (Cobb 2001). Bill Jenkins (chapter 8) presents findings of research carried out with a group of hospice chaplains in the United Kingdom. Both Millard's and Jenkins's chapters expand on the theme of mutuality in relationships that seek to offer spiritual care.

In chapter 9, Paul Beirne explores a particular aspect of palliative care experience—the encounter between different belief and value systems as individuals meet in caring relationships. Finally, John Paver (chapter 10) gathers up a number of themes from the other chapters as he reflects upon his experience as chaplain, educator, and cancer sufferer.

The care-givers' voices in this part reflect the Christian tradition, as well as the changes that are taking place for most practitioners who have a religious allegiance. While committed to a particular tradition these care-givers show openness to other traditions and approaches. They are not interested in reasserting a religious dominance of spiritual concerns: indeed, they critique religious approaches as well as question contemporary approaches that neglect religious resources or dismiss pastoral skills.

REFERENCE

Cobb, M. 2001, *The Dying Soul: Spiritual Care at the End of Life*, Open University Press, Buckingham.

6

It's the Way My Spirit Speaks

Maggie May

THE ILLNESS STORY

I was first diagnosed with malignant melanoma seventeen years ago. I remember with acute clarity the way my sentence was pronounced. The words still echo in slow motion—'Clarke's level 4—Malignant Melanoma'. This small, dark spot on my lower leg could spread insidiously and fatally throughout my body via my lymphatic system.

My world turned, mortality was acknowledged, there was a shift in perspective on all levels. My life changed forever.

But why me?

I thought I was handling life well enough. I ate health foods, whole foods, was making an effort to be aware, physically, intellectually, emotionally, and spiritually. I cared about other people and did my share of marching for moratoriums, demonstrating for causes—to save old buildings, save the planet, and stop the war. (One tends to make value judgments when looking for cause and effect—anything to grasp onto.) Perhaps there had been a mistake?

There had not been. The situation was alarming, the operation scheduled for the following day. Then came the other practical implications, disablement, and rehabilitation. The new and strange powerlessness of being dependent on others, and the big 'Will I be all right?' question.

At this point I should sketch a brief outline of my personal history. I was born in 1944 in Warrnambool, country Victoria. I was the eldest of seven children and my mother was preoccupied looking after her bedridden mother in the nearby town, so the halcyon days of my childhood were spent with my father's parents on their beautiful farming property. Those days were

filled with adventure, endless discussion, the full indulgence and uncon-
ditional love of both grandparents. This closeness may have made it more
difficult for me to relate to my natural parents.

I left home to study at art college, then at teachers' college. My work as a
practising artist combined with my interest in teaching. I was happily married to an architect for ten years. The failure of this marriage brought about a
great loss of confidence and self-esteem. After psychological help and an
intense time absorbed in my artwork I regained myself.

My first melanoma appeared around this time. It had been caused by
exposure to the sun. Diagnosis and treatment were strictly medical matters.
The symptom was cut out. The district nurse thought there was not much
hope, but showed me how to monitor my lymph nodes for further growths.
I sensed then, as I do now, that the symptom could be the beginning of the
cure—that the healing process was more complex, and that it involved my
whole being. Seventeen years ago a holistic approach was considered to be an
act of defiance against Western medical practice: 'There is no quantifiable
evidence to support it.' I remember feeling at odds when I tried to discuss a
dietary approach with an oncologist. Now there is at least a dialogue about
food and cancer.

How did I cope?

There is no doubt in my experience that the stigma of cancer sets one
aside. To stretch a veneer of normality over the chasm of uncertainty requires
effort, physically and mentally. I had to dress differently, even for swimming,
to compensate for the visibly wide incision in my lower leg, cover up against
the sun, reschedule out-of-door activities, and learn to walk without a limp.
Emotionally, it was more difficult. I felt *other* from the majority of healthy
society. Even the simple daily greeting of 'Hi, how are you?' could be a loaded
question, requiring careful response. How was I? All right, I hoped. But if the
question was avoided, then I knew 'they' did not care.

I found that being open to help was difficult, compounded by feeling
insecure and vulnerable. I did not want sympathy, negativity, or curiosity—
I was not sure what parts of conflicting advice I could trust, or where to find
help and support that did not have hidden agendas. I was lucky to have a lifeforce that wanted to be well, and the resource of my art.

Consequently, as an extension of my interests I found strength through
poetry, literature, music, and images. In particular I remember reading
Proust's *Remembrance of Things Past*, the poetry of Cavafy, Neruda, Robert
Graves, Ezra Pound, and listening to the later works of Beethoven—all great

affirmations of the human spirit. My sisters' kindness and care was also wonderful, providing help and nourishment.

My recovery was positive and I was grateful to be alive. The experience had brought living daily into sharp focus. I gained confidence as I got through the three monthly, six monthly, then yearly checkups, with no evidence of growth or spread.

Five years into the clear I met Dennis, an Australian artist who was restoring a folly in north Wales. We formed a strong partnership. I moved to Wales, and we had two children.

Two years later, and seven years after my original melanoma, while I was visiting Australia, I found another small nodule growing beside the original site. It was removed and tested malignant. Again, it was a devastating experience, compounded by my feeling of irresponsibility for having had children. However, I felt I had chosen a partner wisely: younger than me, capable, outdoorish, and extremely healthy, someone dependable now that my health was, again, precarious. We returned to Wales, ever mindful of the precious and temporary nature of life. Once again, my artwork provided a focus for me to make sense of my situation. It was a vehicle in which my interior and exterior worlds connected—or so I thought.

During the next five years life revolved around folly restoration, the children, and local community events, as well as trips to anywhere that could satisfy Dennis's passion for collecting old and antiquarian books. My drawings reflected darkness, threat, protectiveness, hope and beauty, fragility, and a delicate peace.

Nothing could have prepared me for what came next. Early in 1998 Dennis, aged 49, was diagnosed with bowel cancer and liver metastases, another shattering moment that stretched out in vivid slow motion. For someone so full of life, who had so much to live for, the prospect of death was incomprehensible. For Dennis to recognise and prepare for death would have, in his mind, been inviting death itself. So our lives were patterned by the stressful cycle of long-distance travel to hospitals in England, endless waiting rooms, lost CT scans, muddled readings, chemotherapy, hair loss, and false hopes.

As Dennis's cancer developed it progressed to his brain. I would like to think of this as a kindness that allowed him to pass more gently through the transition. He died at home in March 1999 after a year's struggle. The network of support, the local doctor, district nurses, Macmillan nurses (Humphreys-Bartley 2001), palliative care nurses, the priest, and dear friends could not have been more helpful and compassionate. They allowed him to reclaim some of the dignity stripped from him by the nature of the disease and periods of hospitalisation. They made his last wish possible—the peace of dying at home in his chosen environment.

It is too sad and too hard to say any more, except to share an experience I had shortly after Dennis's death.

Early one morning I was given a realisation. The thick pitchpine shutters of my bedroom window had been left open to catch the spring dawn. A voice as clear and silent as the light said, 'His spirit is on Bardsey.' I repeated the words, then realised what they meant. Bardsey is an island off the coast of Wales, where many saints are believed to be buried. I do not think Dennis had ever visited there. The event was extraordinary because it seemed clearly to be a thought that I did not manifest, nor that I could have anticipated. Bardsey is, however, a perfect resting place, among the saints, among the elements. And for me it added a fitting dimension to my understanding and resolution of his life and death.

Subsequently, the children and I decided to return to Australia, to enable us to feel the security of belonging to our wider family of grandparents, aunts, uncles, cousins, and friends.

If my melanoma recurrences have anything to do with fear and stress, then you will have correctly predicted that my third occurrence manifested itself soon after we arrived. This time I was fortunate to receive a more informed diagnosis; with greater knowledge, technical advances, and caring support the experience of hospitalisation and aftercare was much less alienating.

Up until now I thought I was able to access my inner self, enabling a dialogue that could both instruct and heal. My recent illness has provided me with an opportunity to reflect in another way on my story of illness and the way it is linked with my story as an artist.

THE ARTIST'S STORY

I have always preferred to express myself visually. Art school reinforced and encouraged this preference, as well as providing the necessary technical skills. Over the past thirty years I have worked with a variety of media and exhibited regularly. My work as an artist is primarily communication rather than personal statement, that is, what I create, I exhibit. Only once have I decided that a series was more therapy and self-indulgence than communication. That work was recycled and never shown.

Nevertheless, I am aware that what I attempt to communicate through my work is intensely autobiographical. My art offers representations of the world seen through the lens of myself. My drawings and sculptures are observations of my everyday environment, sifted through time and memory. They are introspective—sometimes just marks that represent feelings. I make images in series. Gathering information, distilling, reworking, refining—one process feeds off the other towards an endpoint that may in turn become a new starting point. I understand creativity as positive rather than destructive or negative. My art interprets, cherishes, and preserves the world—it does not attempt to demonise or deconstruct it.

The content of my work has not changed appreciably with my illness. The central images with which I continue to work were already firmly established, based in and inspired by the natural environment and its parallels in the human psyche, the echoes and reverberations that are held within our experience and possibly collective memory. One recurring theme is the impact of the elements on the surface of forms, revealing their history through their building up and wearing away. Another is personal and universal juxtaposition, with its overlays of energies, patterns and rhythms. There are often references to light and shadow, strength and fragility, delicacy and threat, life and death. My large drawings use a variety of media to explore symbolically these themes. Smaller drawings provide more detailed investigative studies.

It is only recently, through an intersubjective exploration of my work, that I have recognised that art has been for me a place to record and deposit my experiences, but not a means for reviewing, resolving, or reconstructing what I have represented. My art is a story of myself, but it has not been consciously available to me. The layers of information were recorded, but I did not have the skills to access them on a personal level. This in no way detracts from or interferes with their aesthetic integrity, but illustrates the possibilities of bringing another mode of expression or understanding to bear. The intersubjective method has made me an interpreter—as well as the maker—of my own work.

The method operates from the premise that the creative process is a way of knowing. Works of art are representations of knowledge; by attending closely using a phenomenological method, further layers of meaning can be accessed and expressed (Lett 1998). It is an important tool for all involved in the pursuit of self-knowledge, whether through therapy, spiritual companioning, or creative projects. Companionship is a fundamental, if not essential, aspect of intersubjective exploration, that is, a trusted person is needed to support, facilitate, and share the exploration. In my case my companion was a relative, skilled in creative arts therapy.

The drawing with which we chose to work at depth was 'Wind of Thorns' (Figure 6.1). Here the central motif of worn and patinated sea shells is surrounded by a collaged circle. A spiky form hovers above. These shells, collected on one of our family walks, are metaphors for our life, placed in an act of symbolic protectiveness.

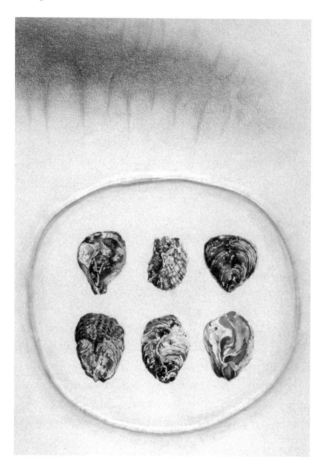

Figure 6.1 'Wind of Thorns'

'Wind of Thorns' comes from the period after my second melanoma but before Dennis's diagnosis. It was a time when there should not have been clouds on the horizon. The drawing developed in three distinct phases, although this was not premeditated: as remarked earlier, one process led to another. My original intention was to record the beautiful colours and patterns of the shells I found in the sparkling icy water on a bright winter's morning as we walked along the Welsh coastline and to preserve the associated memory of our experience as a family. The second stage became a necessary addition because the shells appeared vulnerable. To symbolically protect them I encircled them with papier mâché, not an illusion, but an actual three-dimensional form made from layers of tissue, string, and glue. Then, not being able to leave well enough alone, during a third phase of drawing I added the dark threatening cloud and the thorny spikes.

My initial understanding of the drawing was that it recorded our experience and, perhaps, commented on the delicate nature of our pleasure, of life, and of our environment. The intersubjective process of interpretation began by looking afresh at this work and describing what I saw. My companion recorded these words, inviting me to identify the focus of interest and the places or features to which my eye returned. We then selected independently from this to record the words that appeared to us to be keys, grouping and arranging them in patterns. From this we made individual responses that captured the essence of the drawing.

I made a diagram (figure 6.2) in which the words are categorised into compartments that reflect my personal realm.

Using the same word source my companion offered her response in a series of haiku.

The tide gone out left
Bright wet fissures on hard sand.
In this brightness, shells.

Traceries of holes,
Shells ... built up and worn back down
Lives made visible!

Cold pain spikes down but
My attention turns around,
Finds balance, resolve.

Shell at the centre,
Less worn, beautiful, balanced ...
I return to this.

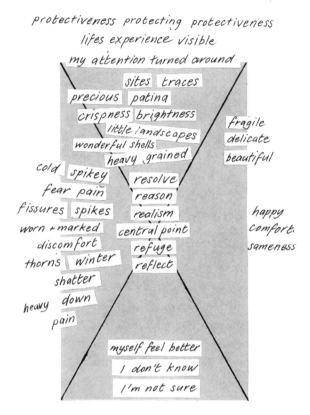

Figure 6.2 protectiveness protecting protectiveness

As we worked backwards and forwards between the visual and verbal representations patterns emerged, and I began to see quite clearly how the content of my work paralleled passages in my life. I could also see how I had been working and reworking particular themes, ritualistically using them as a way of making my life secure. With this insight came new possibility. Now I was able to make connections that could resolve and reconstruct my story. An example of this is the essence statement that emerged spontaneously as we reflected on the project represented in my collected works of art, 'It's the way my spirit speaks.'

Without the deep trust I had in my companion's sensitivity, perception, and skill in interpretation this process could not have unfolded. The exploration was genuinely helpful, yet, paradoxically, it was help I was scarcely aware of needing, nor would I have known where to go for it even had I been aware of need. Because the exploration was informal, and carried out within an existing relationship, it took place without the expectations or inhibitions

I associate with organised therapeutic activities. Through it I have learnt a new skill that I can call upon to enhance my creative activity. The availability of the new skill does not change or inhibit my creative process, but it does allow me to reflect upon it and draw out from it further insights. I become not only the creator but an interpreter of my own work, and through this learning continue to develop as an artist who, I have now realised, can explore the sacred within everyday life.

WEAVING THE STORIES

Reflecting on the strands of my story it is evident that my expression through my art has given me a sense of purpose, a touchstone, and has been a great companion, especially in times of crisis. I have discovered that an illness if engaged can focus and inform the life quest.

In my case, having my life project as an artist in place before encountering my illness provided a substantial and continuous resource. Illness brought priorities—urgency, and a greater understanding of the human condition—and a shift in perception.

I have found within myself strength to endure and transcend my illness. It is not a resource I have developed intentionally; it is simply there. Even so, it must be drawn upon, nurtured, and directed. Here, my art is the essential tool, putting me in touch with the inner strength that keeps me going. My vocation holds me in place, connecting the depths of my spirit with the world in which I live.

Through my encounter with illness I know there is a lifeforce greater than my physical dimension, and that the dialogue between paint and paper and myself contains the intangible—call it the creative—force. I had an orthodox religious upbringing in a conservative Protestant Christian tradition and, perhaps ironically, this has served to obscure any connections between the spirituality of my work and my religious heritage. The religious ways of knowing to which I was subjected were at odds with my sensitivities: words and music seemingly lacked the inwardness I needed, and images—or at least images that could inspire and compel—were absent. My connections with religious traditions are now mediated through culture—the art and music that inspire and nurture me.

I realise the significance of companions on the journey, the need to draw on the creativity of others, including the great creative mentors I've mentioned in my illness story, to nurture the creativity in my self and the need to share the illness load. The spiritual communities in which I participate and that hold me accountable are informal. The most consistent is the intangible community of art, where the music of Tavener connects me to the orthodox liturgy, or the paintings of Morandi, which connect me with a world of distilled poetic imagery. The essential connections are established through the lens of my art—the hidden beauty of natural objects and the ways in which they reveal our human finitude and vulnerability, yet also the enduring impulse of care and love that holds us all. Even without my illness I made these connections, but living with melanoma and living through Dennis's dying have sharpened my awareness of how quite ordinary objects and events can become transparent to the spirit that surrounds and permeates our existence. This perception, mediated through a reflective process which, for me, involves creating works of art, sets up responsive resonances in my own spirit and creates community with those others, living and dead, whose words, music, and images encourage and challenge me to attend to my spirit's voice.

REFERENCE

Humphreys-Bartley, L. 2001, 'Macmillan nurses' in G. Howarth & O Leaman (eds), *Encyclopedia of Death and Dying*, Routledge, London, pp. 292–3.

Lett, W. 1998, 'Researching experiential self-knowing', *The Arts in Psychotherapy*, vol. 25, no. 5, pp. 331–42.

7

Facing the Situation

Regina Millard

In this chapter I discuss spirituality, spiritual issues, and spiritual care in palliative care, drawing on my personal experience and practice as a pastoral carer in the field of community-based palliative care.

The role of the pastoral care worker is to listen to the stories of the patients or carers and the stories of team members about their patients and carers with ears attuned to the soul. The pastoral carer may respond directly to the patient or carer as part of the pastoral care role or act as a resource person to facilitate and support a team member's response. The pastoral carer is available to reflect with palliative care team members on their efforts to provide spiritual care and help the team bring spiritual issues into focus when they may otherwise escape notice. The pastoral care worker's role also extends to mobilising, supporting, or coaching resource people in the wider community to provide spiritual support to a dying person or to his or her carers.

It has already been noted that there can be some confusion about the use of the words 'pastoral' and 'spiritual'. In this chapter pastoral care is used as an umbrella term encompassing spiritual care and religious care. The pastoral carer then is the one who listens for and responds to a person's spiritual or religious needs. The challenge for the pastoral carer is to actively support and encourage all care team members to recognise spirituality as integral to the holistic care we offer.

MY STORY

I have been a Roman Catholic Sister of Charity for thirty-three years. The Irish Sisters of Charity pioneered hospice care in the early 1800s in Ireland

and the Australian Sisters of Charity began the first hospice in Australia in 1890, the Sacred Heart Hospice in Darlinghurst, New South Wales. Care of the dying has been a part of my Order's mission from its beginning. I was educated in the Roman Catholic school system prior to the Second Vatican Council and began my training to become a Sister of Charity when the Council was in session in 1965. After I made my religious profession as a Sister of Charity in 1967, I became a registered nurse and practised nursing for more then twenty years. Religion and religious practice had been important in my family life, and so it continued to be in my chosen vocation. I felt I never imposed religion on people, but as a religious sister caring for the sick there was an expectation that I would also be helping patients prepare their souls for the next life. Many patients and staff saw me as having a religious pastoral care role simply because I was a religious sister, readily identified by the way I was dressed. If religious care was needed, I felt at home providing it. To think of spirituality being anything other than a person's religion did not enter my consciousness at this time.

Eventually, I changed direction professionally and moved from nursing to pastoral care. With the primary source for the practice of this pastoral care being biblical, and the commonly held image of pastoral care being that of Jesus the Good Shepherd, it was a comfortable shift for me to make. Healing, guiding, supporting, and reconciling were all contained in this shepherding role. But this comfortable religious understanding was to be challenged.

Exposure to the clinical pastoral education movement in the 1970s began to slowly change and broaden my understanding of pastoral care. Pastoral care now encompassed many other ways in which people sought meaning in their lives; religious belief was not the only way. The broader view of spirituality became clearer to me; I began to see spirituality as unique as the individuals who embody it. Belonging to a particular religious belief system no longer held the monopoly on meaning or spirit.

This was a major shift for me. It did not mean I had to stop being myself, or abandon my faith tradition, or stop responding to people's religious needs. It did, however, require me to integrate traditional and new learnings and open myself to the many ways people seek and find meaning in their lives. My pastoral formation moved from a model of religious pastoral care to an incarnational pastoral care, grounded in shared human experience and shared searching. The healing, guiding, supporting, and reconciling, which seemed exclusive to religious shepherding, now took on the broader objectives of healing, guiding, supporting, reconciling, nurturing, liberating, and empowering people in all aspects of their lives (Lartey 1997). The task now was to be a shepherd of the soul.

Other images of pastoral care emerged, such as wounded healer, soul friend, companion, and guide. I grew to be both firm and flexible in my own faith tradition while at the same time affirming and celebrating the plurality and diversity of another's spirituality. Pastoral care of people now assumed a mutual relationship, not an authoritarian one by virtue of my religious profession. Other aspects besides religious faith also constituted my own personal spirituality. I became aware that while at times my formal religious identity as a Sister of Charity stimulated some people to verbalise spiritual and religious concerns it had the opposite effect for others of inhibiting discussion, especially in today's secularised society. Because of this, I usually meet people unidentified as a professed religious. As a relationship develops, this aspect of my identity may be revealed—or it may not. The comfort of the other is paramount.

The Catholic Health Association of the United States (1990), in a document on quality assurance and pastoral care, stated that pastoral carers can no longer hide behind the clerical shield, as people today ask not only for compassion, but competency, a competency whose training, specialisation and certification processes supersede ordination or religious formation in and by itself. My journey continues to be a spiritual one, in the sense of spirituality being that which shapes meaning and purpose for my life. The journey over these years has been both challenging and enriching, and continues to be so as I open myself to the experience of accompanying dying people and their carers, listening for their expression of their souls in the conversations I have with them.

WHAT DOES IT MEAN TO BE SPIRITUAL AND HOW IS THAT EXPRESSED BY THE DYING?

The most basic human spiritual longings are for love, belonging, and acceptance. Spirituality—and its expression—is subject to individual understanding. When talking about the spiritual, soul and spirit are often used interchangeably. The word 'spirit' comes from the Latin *spiritus* meaning 'breath', the source of human life. May (1982) suggests that soul and spirit are not 'things' to believe or not to believe, but rather ways of describing existence—soul indicating essence and spirit indicating fundamental energy. Lennox (1998) reports Michael Leunig, a popular Australian spiritual cartoonist and writer, as saying that spirit is the impulse towards life, the Eros in a person leaping forward. Soul, according to Leunig, refers to something long-suffering, where meanings are made and where there is a sense of the eternal, a sense that we are more than our bodies and minds, that our death is not the most important thing, nor our life. The spiritual then is what people may identify as their reason for being or that which provides meaning to their existence. It is something that gives coherence and direction to life. People will give expression to their soul in many ways; thus spirituality can help people transcend their present situations and live more fully in the present, as the following case studies suggest.

> Jerry, aged 68, married with three adult children and about to become a grandfather for the first time, wrote these words as he was dying of mouth cancer.
>
> What matters to me now is the quality of the experiences I have with people and particularly with my partner, my children, and my intimate friends. Like going for a walk around the block at 7 a.m. makes me feel connected rather than being surrounded by people who want to help me, by protecting me, doing things for me, etc. ... I need to feel I am part of things, diminished though it may be. I am my Spirit—my life, all the wonderful sharings I've had with people ... I want to celebrate with the people I love, my life, as well as my death. I still want them to be open to me as I'd like to be with them. Sometimes this will be pleasant, sometimes painful. Love to me is sharing all of this ...

Spirituality may be influenced by a person's culture, sex, race, family environment, or moral stance. We all have a spirituality of some kind. A person's soul may find expression through the body, the mind, feelings, and creative activities. In whatever way it is expressed, the search for meaning and purpose is a common and fundamental spiritual quest. We are more aware now that what is spiritual is not necessarily religious.

> Maggie, aged 42, divorced, no children, has always had creative gifts, but as she is faced with her death she has a heightened desire and sense of urgency to use these gifts for her own wellbeing. She always wanted to move to the country, have her own garden, and spend time drawing and painting. This brings her life. She has a close circle of friends who want to be there for her and she wants to take every opportunity to be with them. She wants to be free of the debilitating relationship she has with her mother in order to pursue what has always been meaningful to her. She decided to seek professional help to do this.

Spirituality is a path that takes us from the superficial to the depths, or from the outer person to the inner person (Fox 1991). When a person is dying this movement can take place very quickly as people ask, 'What does this all mean for me?' Such a spiritual quest becomes religious when a person begins to identify a relationship with the 'Ultimate Spirit' or 'Mystery of life' (May 1982). This often happens for dying people faced with the mystery of what is beyond death: there can be a deep desire to be connected to something or someone beyond themselves.

> Gary, aged 49, married with two young children and dying of motor neurone disease, wrote his own eulogy, in which he expressed the religious aspect of his spiritual quest.
>
> Did I ask God why? Yes, but it was never a burning issue. Rather, I was guided by the question what can I learn from all this? Learn I did, but maybe not enough. In the last few years of my life I did search for meaning in all this. My journey took me along many paths of discovery. I delved into the Bible, fundamentalist Christian literature, Eastern philosophy and many treatises on suffering and evil. Along the way I became richer in my beliefs … Did I actually find meaning in all this? No, in a religious sense it made no sense, except for the belief in eternal salvation through Christ's death on the cross …

While many people today are consciously on spiritual journeys of some kind, others would not identify themselves as spiritual. Yet, when physical existence is threatened by the prospect of death and physiological needs for survival can no longer be met, spirituality, whether already formed or previously unrecognised, can become a source of meaning, hope, strength, and transcendence.

LISTENING IS ESSENTIAL

What is pastoral listening? How is it different to other forms of listening? Robert Twycross, the English pioneer of palliative care, suggests (1995) that the spiritual dimension of a person is what holds together the physical, psychological, and social dimensions of our lives. Total care of a person, then, involves all four dimensions. The pastoral care worker, through good listening and companioning, can assist people to become more aware of their own values, hopes, and longings as they search to make sense or meaning of their illness. Thus they can express their soul and use their spirituality to face their present situations and, in some, cases transcend them.

In contemporary palliative care services, pastoral carers usually operate in clinically organised settings. Their listening, however, is that of a pastoral companion, or a soul companion, not that of a clinical assessor (Moran 1996). Moran notes that the Greek word *psyche* means both mind and soul, so it is easy to see how these two concepts can be confused in practice. Psychologists and psychiatrists use 'psyche' to mean 'mind', priests and spiritual directors to mean 'soul'. Both are really speaking about the spiritual dimension of the human being, but there is a distinction between the two intellectual traditions. One is 'philosophical-theological' and the other 'psychological' (Moran 1996). It is the former that contributes to the identity of pastoral carers.

While palliative care professes a holistic approach to care, the dual forces of mainstreaming and fiscal constraint are contributing to clinical dominance of the field. In clinical settings, spiritual care is in danger of becoming routinised along with all other disciplines by an emphasis upon standardised determinations of needs, goals, care plans, and measurable outcomes. It seems to be the trend in some palliative care services to absorb the spiritual dimension of care into psychosocial services. It is assumed that anyone with life experience can address spiritual issues, that the terms 'spiritual' and 'pastoral' need not be included explicitly in the language of multidisciplinary care, and that professional pastoral care can be dispensed with or substituted for by community providers on demand. However, if belief is important for the person and is opened up for discussion and reflection, it is important that the person's needs are met through someone competent and comfortable with having belief systems—or God—as the focus of the relationship. Further, beneath everyday words a trained person can often discern complex philosophical and theological questions that are being raised (Millard 1999). This competence cannot be assumed of every team member, as many may have no training in pastoral listening or pastoral practice at all. By ignoring pastoral skills we risk spiritual care being reduced to psychological care. Indeed, I find myself constantly asking for the words 'pastoral' or 'spiritual' to be added when I hear them being omitted. The omission denies, even if unconsciously, the spiritual dimension of the care we offer.

We have all experienced the negative effect of people who do not listen and the positive feeling gained from people who listen well. To be able to listen and hear another's soul is a particular gift and requires particular skill. Along with listening, the gift of insight or discernment is required in order to recognise the soul when it is revealed. Those offering pastoral care require listening ability coupled with insight. Clinical pastoral education and reflective practice are ways that listening and discernment can be brought into focus for the pastoral carer. In discussing the routinisation of spiritual care Walter (1997) suggests that if all staff are to be open to offering spiritual care, how are they to know when to stop busily doing and just *be* with the patient? The ethos of nursing involves getting through the work and the ethos of medicine involves being in control, but the ethos of spiritual care entails entering into the vulnerability of listening and being, and of not necessarily having answers. Saunders (1998) says it is a 'question of time, and timing: a readiness on the part of all staff to stop and listen at the moment this particular area of pain is expressed, and to stay with it'.

Pastoral listening is distinctive in style, distinguishable from that of a counsellor, therapist, or spiritual director. There are several features that characterise it. The pastoral ear

- seeks to hear the other as a unique person
- vigilantly and constantly listens to one's own self before listening to the other so that there is minimal possibility of confusion between the inner world of the listener and the inner world of those seeking help
- is one that is provided by a person who has a background of knowledge of professionals who could gain further access to a person's inner world should it be needed.

Pastoral listening, then, centres on the inner world of the human being (Moran 1996). The listening of the social worker, the nurse, the doctor, in their various realms of care, are all means by which the person builds on or adjusts to their inner world. Because of this, it is vital that all professions listen well.

PASTORAL CARE AND THE PALLIATIVE CARE TEAM

Pastoral care in palliative care aims to support a good death through holistic practice, assuming that meaning and purpose can be discovered or reaffirmed in the face of suffering and death. The goal is to help people live with the inevitable uncertainties of life-threatening illness, to discover inner resources for dealing with ambivalence or anxiety, and to support them as they struggle to review the meaning of their lives and in making realistic choices (Rumbold 1998).

There is a great deal of confusion in the general community—as well as within some palliative care agencies—about what pastoral care has to offer people. Many pastoral carers themselves find it difficult to express succinctly the range of their interests and interventions, in part because these are strongly influenced by context. In community palliative care, for example, the person is not captive in a bed waiting for what we have to offer. They are in their own homes, in control of their own environment. A community of people who, in a variety of ways, can offer support and nourish spirituality surrounds them. The pastoral carer needs to be aware of these supports and help to mobilise them with and for the patient and carers. So the question may be asked, how does pastoral care enter or begin?

In the service in which I work it is never presumed that the sick person or the carers do or do not need the pastoral care service. A phone call is made to ask if the pastoral care person could come and be introduced to explain what support may be offered from the service involved or the wider community around them. A small leaflet in the admission folder explaining pastoral care stimulates conversation when the visit is made. Control rests with the person and the pastoral carer responds and facilitates care as needed. Sometimes there is instant acceptance because the support offered is needed; others are more tentative and are invited to make contact when they feel ready, while still others refuse outright. All responses are respected. However, unless other team members work with the pastoral carer to clarify the role, the offer of pastoral care can be interpreted solely as an offer of religious support. Many times the response to the offer of pastoral care made by the person assessing and admitting is, 'No thank you, I'm not a churchgoer.'

All team members need to be clear about the breadth of pastoral care, and it is the pastoral carer's responsibility to keep all team members informed about spiritual care. This may be achieved by formal education sessions conducted in time allocated for team education, offering the staff reading material for reflection and discussion, periodically using a case conference in which pastoral care was integral to the person's total care. As the facilitator of spiritual care on the team, help can be given to team members on the spot or whenever the need arises for them to discuss issues of spiritual care. The pastoral carer needs to be constantly alert to ways of raising the profile of spiritual care among team members who, in turn, take it to the community. Hopefully, they too are challenged to have some answer to the question: What is spiritual care and why is it important in palliative care?

Clergy are often involved in pastoral care in palliative care, but not all clergy are comfortable with people facing death, nor with the debilitation of disease. Recently, when I offered to contact clergy for two dying people, both refused. Each felt their minister was uncomfortable with them and could not talk to them, either about their illness or their dying. As a result, they themselves felt uncomfortable and frustrated, hindered rather than helped. This illustrates the need some people have for their clergy to be more than someone supporting their religious faith. Many clergy are not educated to look for spiritual needs in the broad sense, nor do they have the time needed to explore complex spiritual issues. If a person tells me they are in contact with their particular minister or priest, as pastoral carer I will usually make contact with them to introduce myself and ask if they would like me to keep in contact with them over the time of the person's illness. In this way, there is the possibility of dialogue with them about the broader spiritual issues and an opportunity for mutual support and learning. I acknowledge, however, that there are many helpful and generous clergy who make themselves available and are most sensitive to dying people. Pastoral care in palliative care gives full support to any relationship that contributes to a person's ongoing care.

WHAT DOES PASTORAL CARE IN PALLIATIVE CARE OFFER?

Relationship

Pastoral care offers the person in palliative care a relationship where spiritualities and meanings can meet. As mentioned earlier, this relationship is based on a way of listening that is distinctly pastoral and can identify the soul speaking. Often, the pastoral listening leads into a conversation about forgiveness, love, and hope, language not usually found in counselling or therapy. This is illustrated by Pauline, in her seventies, and close to death.

> Pauline had more time than most after her initial diagnosis of cancer. Our relationship began early in her diagnosis, and trust grew. She shared with me what she later referred to as her deep, dark secret—guilt about the breakdown of her first marriage. She felt responsible. Her adult children of this marriage were aware of this but could not relieve her pain. As her death drew closer she wanted to ask forgiveness of her first husband and once more to express her love for him. This topic came up many times in my visits with Pauline. She expressed the comfort she felt to have someone who was not family to listen to her and to support her as she revisited these feelings and sought ways to forgive and be forgiven.

Supporting realistic hope and sharing in the developing of hope is a major part of spiritual care of the dying. Some practitioners, however, can engender false hope, which can lead to despair.

> Bonnie, in her seventies, was undergoing extensive chemotherapy when she told me that her doctor said that if she persevered with the treatment it would get rid of her cancer. She put so much hope in him. She came to the end of her treatment feeling desperately ill and facing death. She felt cheated and angry.

A minister is often called in when nothing more can be done for the person medically. A shift occurs from hope in recovery to hope in immortality. This in itself is not necessarily bad, but it equates medicine with life and religion with death (Rumbold 1986). A vital part of helping people to hope is the work of clarification and reflection, which enables the dying person to resolve emotional conflicts. Without such resolution, the dying person is less likely to engage with questions of meaning and purpose that can lead to hope and transcendence. The issue of hope in the face of dying is a complex one and requires experience from the person offering spiritual care. It also requires time. Bonnie was deprived of the time she needed to adjust her hope.

Time and continuity within a pastoral relationship are essential for developing trust and supporting hope. Because of this, early referral to palliative care is desirable, but because communication between some oncology and palliative care practitioners remains poor, early referral to palliative care does not always happen readily. The focus of care continues to be primarily medical, with the reasoning that this is necessary to foster hope for life. But it may be false hope. More realistic hopes could be sought in such things as feeling better tomorrow, finding daily or weekly satisfactions, leaving something of lasting value to others, or a hope to transcend or survive present pain (Kellehear 1999).

Early referral is essential to address these hope issues. One Melbourne oncologist employs a pastoral care worker in his rooms and in the day oncology service he attends. This worker is available as close as possible to diagnosis and able to work with people at their most vulnerable moment—a rare and encouraging practice. To be available early gives the person a chance to express feelings. It also provides the support necessary to make informed choices about his or her ongoing care and management. Such an approach is consistent with a health-promoting palliative care (Kellehear 1999), which places the illness prevention approach of general health promotion alongside the illness management approach of palliative care. Health-promoting palliative care provides education and information on health, dying, and death, as well as providing social support from a variety of settings. It also encourages interpersonal problem solving. Many practitioners now acknowledge that a lot of useful work with seriously ill people might be done earlier in their illness rather than later. Without such a shift, pastoral care will probably be limited to a supportive role on the margins of palliative care programs, failing to make its significant creative contribution (Rumbold 1998).

In my experience, most referrals to community palliative care do not come early enough, admittedly sometimes because the patients themselves do not want it. The thought of being admitted to a palliative care service can be very confronting and frightening. However, there are now occasions when a person with terminal illness is admitted to the community palliative care program for pastoral care only. For some this is a way of coming to terms with what lies ahead for them, allowing them to prepare for a peaceful death, to seek support for their sometimes fragile hope, and explore ways to cope. Support from a person outside the family can be helpful through relieving the burden on the carers. Such early referrals allow the person and pastoral carer time to get to know each other and for the relationship to develop. From this relationship the movement from the superficial to the depths, from the outer to the inner person, may occur, with support (Fox 1991). Early referral for pastoral care may also influence how the person—and his or her carers—approach further treatment decisions, where the person wishes to die, and, ultimately, the way in which death itself takes place.

Listening

Pastoral care offers a listening presence that attends to the soul of the other. In their inner world many may experience spiritual pain—a lack of hope, purpose, meaning, and, for some, lost connections to family or community (Saunders 1988). Often the initial desire on meeting a person with a life-threatening illness who has this emotional and spiritual pain and confusion is to want to fix it or take it away. Pastoral carers in palliative care can be tested when they find themselves feeling this way. Fundamental to pastoral listening and relationship is the understanding that all people are responsible for their own unique inner world. The aim of pastoral listening is to assist the speaker to take this responsibility seriously. To do so means that pastoral listeners must recognise their limits and be clear about who indeed is the best suited to help a person come to terms with what is needed (Moran 1996).

Maggie, cited earlier, spoke to me many times about her painful childhood and, arising from this situation, the intolerable relationship with her mother (now 80). She has lived with this to a certain extent and got on with her life. Now, in her changed life situation, Maggie finds that relationship more painful than ever to speak about and when she does the speaking now is always accompanied by uncontrollable crying. She has undergone therapy for a few years—being 'on the couch', she called it—but now, with a life-threatening illness, she is seeking to develop her spiritual life in order to gain some peace. I helped her as far as I could but, ultimately, dealing with her mother was her responsibility. I offered referral to a palliative care psychiatrist who specialised in family relationships.

Pastoral care embraces both giving and receiving. Pastoral care does not impose answers to another's questions. If the soul of a person can be nurtured in a mutual way and life be affirmed in the face of death, there may be positive consequences in the quality of life for the dying person. The pastoral care person, through good listening and companioning, can assist people to become aware of their own values, hopes, strengths, and longings, as they search to make sense or meaning of their living and dying. Pastoral care offers a safe place for thoughts and feelings to be expressed and heard.

Ritual

Pastoral care offers opportunity for ritual that is an imaginative and interpretive act through which meaning is expressed and created (Anderson & Foley 1998). Ritual can be very powerful in expressing or creating meaning for the dying person and his or her carers. It can also create a comforting memory for carers after the person's death.

Our lives are a series of unconscious rituals, but there are times when ritual needs to become a conscious act. Rituals can range from a very simple use of symbols, actions, words, or music, to the very complex. It depends totally on what people wish to express. Ritual may be asked for as a rite of passage to transcend one reality to another, for example, from denial to acceptance, letting go of life into death. The pastoral carer is simply the facilitator for the person wanting the ritual. Some rituals may be requested early after diagnosis, others much later.

Joan, aged 54 and close to death, reminisced with me about her life and one particular area in which she felt she was a burden to her husband and daughter because of a depressive illness. She remembered how important her own mother's words and actions were before her death. I asked if she would like to express some of her thoughts and feelings to her husband and daughter in the form of a simple ritual in her home, and to allow them to express theirs with my help. She jumped at the opportunity to be supported in doing this. The ritual consisted of bringing Joan, husband, and daughter together in the comfort of their livingroom. After all was said, I invited husband and daughter to move closer and hold Joan as I read a verse that encapsulated something of what the family had shared. They were then given the opportunity to express what they wanted to express as they continued to hold her near. The ritual brought tears, but it helped them all to attend to the five things of relationship completion described by Byock (1997): I forgive you, forgive me, I love you, thank you, goodbye.

For the team members ritual is also an important part of pastoral care in palliative care. At my place of work a monthly time of reflection for all team members is part of a set monthly team day. Included in this is a time of what I call deflection and reflection. Deflection allows an opportunity to unload feelings and move forward emotionally and psychologically in a supportive atmosphere. Reflection encourages the team to slow down, be still, and look inward. The reflection segment includes a ritual and offering of the names of those who have died in the past month. Having time to reflect on how the patients and carers have touched our lives can help us to gently hold the experiences, while at the same time move us on to those awaiting care. Facilitating ritual and education about the place of ritual in our lives is very much part of what pastoral care contributes. It is a way of offering spiritual care to the team members.

Bereavement care

Coming to terms with the impending loss of one's life and relationships can sometimes be overlooked in the dying person. The pastoral care person can navigate a passage through this grief, with the person, thereby improving his or her quality of life for the time remaining. Contact with the carers can also prove very helpful in addressing their grief issues as they let go, and in offering referral to support services within the community following the death of the person. Sometimes the relationship is extended into the time of bereavement.

THE IMPORTANCE OF THE PERSONAL JOURNEY

Essential to companioning others on their spiritual journey and listening to their souls is the development of one's own soul's journey. The gap between theoretical insight about the importance of spiritual care in palliative care and personal daily practice needs to be narrowed in order to truly hear another. Pastoral care in palliative care particularly requires some previous contemplation about death and dying and what it all means personally. The effect of death within my own life, how I coped, how I reacted, or what I personally believe about death and beyond can influence the pastoral response—for better or worse.

Pastoral supervision is very valuable in this area of the personal journey. Caring for the spirit of another carries with it the implication of caring for myself and fostering the ability to stay with what is weak and vulnerable in myself and others. Otherwise a great deal of projection onto the other of my ideas, needs, and pain may occur. We ought not underestimate how hard it is to listen and be compassionate. Compassion is difficult because it requires the inner disposition to go with others to the place where they are weak, vulnerable, lonely, and broken. This is not our spontaneous response to suffering. We prefer to flee from it or find a quick cure for it. By keeping busy and feeling relevant we ignore our greatest gift, the ability to be there, listen, and enter into solidarity with another suffering human being (Nouwen 1981).

A wise spiritual companion or some form of supervision—either individual or with colleagues—can enrich and encourage personal daily practice in the palliative care field. It is true that any empathetic, warm, listening human being *may* bring comfort to a dying person, but sensitivity and perception are also important ingredients. Unless we are occupied in our own search for meaning we may not create the climate in which people can be helped to make their own journeys of growth through loss (Saunders 1988). It is equally important to listen for feedback received from people in our care because it gives clues to the what and how of our communication with them. After Pauline's death I received these words from her daughter: 'Mum received great comfort and pleasure from your talks together. You responded so sensitively to her needs and enabled her to confide her deepest thoughts and worries in you. What a great gift to have given her—thank you. The spiritual insights you helped her gain were very precious to her. You gave her a steady base from which to approach her death.'

And these words from Pauline herself, just before her death. 'Thank you for the gift of your presence. You are so fond and so loving as you lead and nurture me through the closing chapters of my life. There is a deep sense of community with you.'

SPIRITUAL ISSUES AND NEEDS IN PALLIATIVE CARE

Human beings are meaning-makers and meaning-seekers with an innate desire to transcend or move beyond situations of hardship or suffering. Examples of this surround us daily through the media or through our own life experiences. Facing a life-threatening illness heralds issues of loss and separation as well as all the fears associated with facing death. It is common to want to move beyond these things and live, because the desire to live is normal.

Finding effective tools for assessing spiritual needs continues to be a challenge for researchers and writers in spirituality. Kellehear (2000) proposed a theoretical model of spiritual needs in palliative care that is multidimensional and arises from different dimensions of spirituality. In the clinical arena this model best describes and organises my personal experiences of pastoral care in palliative care. Spiritual needs are grouped under the following headings:

- situational needs
- moral/biographical contexts
- religious beliefs and ideas.

Kellehear sees these groups as possible sources of transcendence and building blocks for spiritual meaning at a time of illness and distress.

Situational needs arise out of the immediate situation in which people find themselves. For some, this may be at the time of diagnosis, for others, later in the disease process, or just somewhere along the way. It is a time of questioning, both inwardly and outwardly. Changes are taking place in their lives at all levels—physically, socially, emotionally, and spiritually. What does it all mean? What can I expect? What can I hope for? How will this affect my work, my family? How do I keep connected with the world and people? It is at times like this that the person may begin to look for someone to relate to and reflect with. This may be the pastoral care worker or another who can meet the need. For example, some of the needs expressed by Joan (introduced previously) were to

- have some idea how she will die; will her family be protected from a distressing death?

- maintain external, cosmetic appearance even in the presence of a deteriorating body because this was part of defining herself to others
- know, after years of depression, that she was accepted by her family
- make sure her husband had permission to move on with his life after her death and pursue another relationship
- consciously do 'the lasts' with her daughter
- achieve small goals relating to social activity
- reconnect with a dormant religious faith.

Joan, realising her prognosis was poor, wanted someone other than a family member with whom she could reflect and explore these issues. I responded and met with her regularly. The family too were relieved that she had such a person. Her sister commented to me one day, in front of Joan, 'Thank you for helping Joan to be peaceful'.

Moral and biographical needs arise due to the person's decline in health and their impending death. The past can become very vivid when facing death, and particular events may need to be celebrated or reconciled. The present, with its feelings of loneliness, abandonment, helplessness, and impending loss, needs to be lived in and dealt with. The future needs to be looked to with realistic hope.

Some people need to finish unfinished business in order to move on psychologically; they need to right wrongs, ask forgiveness, or heal a relationship. Kellehear describes this category of needs as semireligious in nature but not necessarily approached through a religious dogma or theology. Some are helped by prayer, but they are not necessarily religious. Some people are interested in the next life, but not for theological reasons. Jerry, cited earlier, expressed his needs this way.

> I would like some help for Maria in dealing with the chores—the best help she can be to me is to support me morally and make whatever adjustments she can to deal with this most complex of change. What I need from her is not to be looked after physically but to be there for me psychologically, that is, affirm my ambivalence and help me deal with it. What I find most difficult is feeling abandoned in the sense that everyone has their agenda for me and is too busy dealing with this that they forget, or may forget, that I have an agenda—perhaps muddled, certainly ambivalent, but nonetheless real. Like, one part of me wants to fit in the need to abandon the fight and accept that the end goal is inescapable—of course I know this—but I need to be helped to do this without feeling I'm abdicating my responsibility towards my life. I've fought this for 4 years … I need to feel that I am part of things,

diminished though it may be. I want to share my pleasures and my pains. I don't want to be seen as a stack of pain and nothing else … I would like people to experience with me that my little walk around the block in the morning, my managing a whole glass of Sustagen without losing it all in spluttering and spitting it out, as my little triumphant project … sometimes it is very, very hard to be where I am and it feels lonely and scary. It doesn't take much to trigger that isolation, aloneness in me.

Religious needs usually present overtly. They become heightened when a person is facing a long illness and death. They are often expressed in requests for religious reconciliation and discussions that focus on being forgiven by God. Prayers to invoke God's mercy, grace, and strength or requests for religious rites become frequent.

Joan found great comfort in her refound Christian religion and regretted she gave it up during her life. She wanted to be part of a church community and take part in its rituals again as she approached death. She asked for prayer at the end of each visit; she said it brought her comfort and reconnected her with God in a formal way.

These three groups of needs may coexist in one person at any given time or one set of needs may dominate. Spiritual needs arise out of the human desire to transcend or go beyond the immediacy of suffering in order to find meaning in the experience. The pastoral carer cannot give the meaning being sought, but when spiritual needs are struggling for expression, someone to be there and listen can assist them, so they do not feel alone on a potentially lonely journey.

CONCLUSION

In Australia, given government funding of palliative care, palliative care pastoral practice is more and more in the clinical arena. This poses two major questions:
- How can pastoral care retain its essential character while participating in clinically organised services?
- Who should practise pastoral care? (Rumbold 2000).

The response to the first question lies in extending the focus of pastoral care beyond the clinical approach to a wider community approach. The health promoting palliative care approach, which reframes hospice practice in a public health model, is an exciting way forward for pastoral care practice.

Response to the second question is in acknowledging the place of pastoral care education with its own body of knowledge and the practice that defines it. Pastoral care is a discipline in its own right and ought not be subsumed under psychosocial disciplines. To offer spiritual care to those with a life-threatening illness may take some well-meaning but untrained people into very unfamiliar territory with no guide.

To face physical decline and mortality is perhaps one of the most stressful times in the life of a human being. Spirituality is meant to nurture the inner person at such times and allow meanings and values to be reaffirmed and perhaps find new expression in their changed situation. Spirituality is also meant to sustain people as they confront some of the demons within, which often emerge during times of great stress and impending loss. Not all people have spiritual needs requiring constant attention. The right of the person to reject spiritual care is always respected. The pastoral carer in palliative care is in a unique position to support people's search for meaning as they and their families face life-threatening illness. This is not achieved alone, but is linked with all care-givers, both professional and nonprofessional. The desire in human beings for transcendence is the source of their spiritual experience. To give good spiritual care requires people to recognise that it encompasses all aspects of the person, including their spirit (Kellehear 2000). As care-givers, we need to be more and more aware of our ability to transcend the ordinariness of our everyday lives and to gather meanings in the unseen worlds of the spirit. Only then can we help ourselves or others face the situation of life-threatening illness.

REFERENCES

Anderson, H. & Foley, E. 1998, *Mighty Stories, Dangerous Rituals*, Jossey-Bass, San Francisco.

Byock, I. 1997, *Dying Well—Peace and Possibilities at the End of Life*, Riverhead, New York.

Catholic Health Association of the United States 1990, *Quality Assurance and Pastoral Care: A Development and Implementation Guide*, St Louis, Missouri.

Fox, M. 1991, *Creation Spirituality*, HarperCollins, San Francisco.

Kellehear, A. 1999, *Health Promoting Palliative Care*, Oxford University Press, Melbourne.

—— 2000, 'Spirituality and palliative care: A model of needs', *Palliative Medicine*, vol. 14, pp. 149–55.

Lartey, E. 1997, *In Living Colour: An Intercultural Approach to Pastoral Care and Counselling*, Cassell, London.

Lennox, G. 1998, *In Search of Heroes: Stories of Seven Remarkable Men*, Allen & Unwin, Melbourne.

May, G. 1982, *Will and Spirit*, HarperCollins, San Francisco.

Millard, R. 1999, 'A place of safe harbour', in M. Box & A. Kellehear (eds), *Sink or Swim: Palliative Care in the Mainstream*, Proceedings of the Inaugural Victorian State Conference in Palliative Care, La Trobe University, Melbourne, 10–12 February, Palliative Care Victoria and Palliative Care Unit, La Trobe University, Melbourne, pp. 35–9.

Moran, F. 1996, *Listening: A Pastoral Style*, Dwyer, Sydney.

Nouwen, H. 1981, *The Way of the Heart*, Harper, London.

Rumbold, B. 1986, *Helplessness and Hope: Pastoral Care in Terminal Illness*, SCM Press, London.

—— 1998, 'Pastoral care of the dying', *Palliative Care Today*, vol.14, pp. 10–11.

—— 2000, 'Pastoral care of the dying and bereaved', in A. Kellehear (ed.), *Death and Dying in Australia*, Oxford University Press, Melbourne.

Saunders, C. 1988, 'Spiritual pain', *Journal of Palliative Medicine*, vol.4, no. 3, pp. 29–32.

Twycross, R. 1995, *Introducing Palliative Care*, Radcliffe Medical Press, New York.

Walter, T. 1997, 'The ideology and organisation of spiritual care: Three approaches', *Palliative Medicine*, vol. 11, pp. 21–30.

8

Offering Spiritual Care

Bill Jenkins

This chapter describes some aspects of an exploration of the consequences of offering spiritual care to those who are dying. Insights were gained through indepth interviews with twelve hospice chaplains who were employed as ecumenical chaplains in free-standing hospices across the United Kingdom. These chaplains were ordained in various mainstream Christian denominations. All were recognised as participating members of the hospice team alongside other healthcare practitioners, principally doctors, nurses, counsellors, social workers, and voluntary carers. The chaplains contributed to the holistic multidisciplinary care of terminally ill patients within a context identified as functional rather than religious (Walter 1997).

Each chaplain's experience was mapped using a fixed schedule of questions that allowed the identification of salient and recurring themes in their experience. The schedule included questions about how they became involved in caring for the dying, what kept them involved, what sorts of relationships had developed, what personal issues had arisen, and how these experiences had shaped their self-understanding and their understanding of their religious heritage. All interviews were recorded and transcribed, then analysed using a phenomenological methodology (Jenkins 1997, pp. 1–20).

The majority of chaplains interviewed were found to have been drawn to hospice chaplaincy through previous contact with those who were dying, either through hospital chaplaincy or parish ministry. Something significant about this contact attracted them to this more specialised ministry. Particularly important in this regard was the mutuality of spiritual care—'reciprocal ministry'—where the one offering the spiritual care also became a recipient of care. Following a brief description of some of the recurring themes, this mutuality of caring, given its centrality, is explored in some detail.

RECURRING THEMES

The mystery of death

Being in close and frequent proximity to the profound mystery of death was identified as an important factor for many of the chaplains, one that provides a sense of awe that is not found when working in a parish. One commented, 'I've seen the other side. There is that X factor. The mystery of it all is quite exciting. It is unquantifiable, and there are depths here that you might never touch bottom in all of this' (Jenkins 1997, p. 24). There was no expressed fear of death or dying, rather, there was the commonly expressed experience of a diminishing fear of death experienced in the presence of those who are dying. 'It helps me to think of my demise. I am not afraid to talk of death, especially to the children' (Jenkins 1997, p. 145).

Establishing relationships

In establishing relationship with patients two elements emerged as significant, both of which depend on various diverse factors: the initial reaction of the patient to the chaplain and, once established, the personal needs of both participants.

The chaplains were not backward in acknowledging their own needs. The sense of pleasure, enjoyment, and fulfilment expressed through their caring defines the meeting of a very obvious human need, but one which they saw ought not to dominate or displace the needs of those who were dying. This kind of honesty was also an outstanding feature of their reflections. It was no more evident than when their sense of vocation was discussed, where any self-sacrificial understanding of ministry was overridden by a very nonromantic and pragmatic approach to their calling, a calling that appears to be based much more on perceived value than on any concept of duty or martyrdom. One commented, 'It pays the bills … [and] … there is the fulfilment of being with a family or with the patient, things that are appreciated' (Jenkins 1997, p. 24). Another said frankly, 'I need to be needed.' And yet another, 'It suits my style, my personality' (Jenkins 1997, p. 27). This shift away from the more common understanding of ministry as self-sacrifice has the potential to distance hospice chaplains from the tradition that has formed their ministry; it is an issue worthy of further exploration.

The elements that contribute to the initial contact being established include the capacity to converse, the willingness of the chaplain to listen, and the willingness of the patient to express his or her need. An important factor in initiating and developing the relationship is the willingness of the chaplain to share the vulnerability of the patient. One chaplain said, 'I pop in and pop out, and just become a familiar figure. And then I say who I am. It's a case of developing trust really' (Jenkins 1997, p. 56). The importance of trust cannot be underestimated; trust of the patient in the chaplain and a trust of the chaplain in the openness of the relationship. There is an element of trusting in the moment for both, with the additional constraint of not looking too far forward. The chaplains know that there will be loss and that they may be affected emotionally, but the willingness to enter unreservedly into a relationship, despite these constraints, is essential.

The relationships that develop cannot do so without trust. In their dying, the patients are coming to a point in their lives where uncertainty may be profound and extensive; the need and the capacity to trust, therefore, take on extreme importance. As objects of this trust, those who offer spiritual care can acknowledge the privilege of being trusted, while at the same time see the trust as directed affection. For many patients, however, the chaplain is seen as the representative of the Church and/or of God. It is only in the development of personal relationships that the formality of the role—or the falseness of the various stereotypical images of chaplain—fades away. Then, two people can meet with an awareness of the wholeness that is available in truly sharing their lives.

The directed establishment of the relationship between the chaplain and the patient was seen to be the responsibility of the chaplain, but all chaplains continually referred to their stance as letting the patients 'set the agenda' for the relationship. For example, one commented, 'I make no demands of them. I enquire after them and I let them set an agenda for our meeting' (Jenkins 1997, p. 51). Such a nondirective stance relinquishes control to the other and makes the chaplains vulnerable as they set aside their 'desire to control [their] immediate circumstances or at least avoid being rendered helpless by them' (Rumbold 1986, p. 29). But this nonassertive position allows them to discern the needs of the patient and avoids the imposition of any religious agenda, a stereotype chaplains report having to confront quite frequently. Allowing the patient to set the agenda, and the potential intimacy arising from accepting this, seems to best characterise fulfilling relationships from the perspective of the one offering the spiritual care.

It may be that the yielding of control is something that needs to be incorporated in the caring approach of the chaplain because it mirrors the active dying of the patient. In dying, the patient is, or is becoming, increasingly helpless, losing control. At the same time, in allowing the patient to set the agenda, the chaplain is giving the patient control, at least over part of the situation in which the patient exists. This is more than an opportunity to discern the needs of the patient; it is an overt act of caring.

This is a different relationship to one based on power, where the chaplain is perceived to have, or to represent, the power to make things right for the one who is dying. The chaplains as a body shied away from any such concept. Their emphasis was more directed to sharing, as openly as possible, the concerns that fill the life of the dying person. It is this being present to the other that is of crucial importance. Being a sign of God's presence or of revealing God's presence was seen to be much more important than seeking any verbal expression of conversion or faith.

The intimate relationships that develop involve reciprocity, a striving for individual presence, each to the other. It is clear that such relationships can be transforming for the chaplain, consistent with the view that human beings '… become real human beings, become persons, when they are converted from their subjective assertion and their will to power, to accept the interpellation of the other and look in the face of the other: the victim, the poor, the widow, the orphan, in biblical terms' (Comblin 1990, p. 51). In a similarly radical way, from the perspective of those who offer spiritual care in the hospice, the chaplains look in the faces of the dying and the grieving and they are changed.

Identification and emotional involvement

In the situation where human beings are offering spiritual care to other human beings who are dying, it is highly probable that personal issues will arise for the carers.

Identification with the patient was an issue for these chaplains, particularly if there were shared characteristics such as age and gender. As one commented, 'If things get a bit close to home, and if situations mirror your own situation that's hurt in the past, then it is hard' (Jenkins 1997, p. 85). Emotional involvement was also seen to be an issue, particularly overinvolvement, which might compromise the capacity to offer spiritual care. Identification might be seen to reflect the processes of empathy at work and involvement the processes of sympathy. The personal issues of identification and emotional involvement also point to a common characteristic of the chaplains interviewed; they are not ministers and priests who set themselves apart from the dying people whom they serve, but men and women who are willing to be with others in their desolation, if this is where the relationship has led them.

Identification and involvement cannot be unrestrained; they do have a cost, and it would be unnatural if the chaplains interviewed did not try to minimise that cost, unless of course they had masochistic tendencies or if they fell into the category of 'corpse skulker', the figure who always seems to be going to funerals of acquaintances, and advising others of the time and place (Canetti 1979, p 21). Hospice chaplains are sometimes seen as having such morbid tendencies, but on the evidence gathered here it is a mistaken view, one that perhaps discounts the calling that is evident in the lives of chaplains and the personal fulfilment that is found by them in offering spiritual care to those who are dying.

It was also evident that chaplains do need to defend themselves from painful aspects of their work. This protection of the self implies that the chaplains may not yield total control of the relationships, but neither do they dominate. This was supported, in one of many ways, by their tendency not to insist that there are issues that have to be addressed by those who are dying before their death. However, they did believe that there were issues that ought to be addressed, practical issues such as those of the estate and the funeral, and the resolution of any relational problems, such that an individual might die in peace, knowing that all their affairs are in order. The basis for this belief emerged from their experience that these things are important for people in that they can have a positive effect on the dying, where the individual may feel more at ease knowing that some kind of closure has been achieved.

The desire for closure—for some kind of completeness—is very common and is rarely achieved. Chaplains know this and yet see closure as a hope that they might have for the other. So there is a real tension for the chaplains between the experience of what they have seen as important and the autonomy of the patient. On the part of the chaplains, in recognising this autonomy they are respecting the freedom, the dignity, and the uniqueness of the patient.

This kind of tension illustrates another more general issue for chaplains, who have a specific religious commitment, but who are prepared to offer spiritual care on the patient's terms, within the context defined by the patient's perceived needs and beliefs. It is essential that chaplains do not exclude from their spiritual care those whose beliefs differ from their own. However, the specific nature of the chaplain's own religious commitment may be a prerequisite to developing the inclusive practices that are reinforced through the experience of hospice ministry.

THE LIMITS TO CARING

The world of the chaplains is bounded by their understanding of what it means to offer spiritual care, the needs of the patients, and by their understanding of their own personal limitations. One of these limitations is the limit to caring, which can be understood in two senses. There is the practical limitation of personal presence, which is a limit of time and place. This is seen also as a limit to opportunity and one that relies on the chaplains being able to trust that the needs of individual patients can be met by others, not simply by other chaplains, but by hospice staff, or relatives, or friends.

The other limit is that set by the concept 'professional', the set of common core values that exist within, and describe, a particular ethos that includes personal noninvolvement. This was seen as a limit to personal relationship by all the chaplains in this study and, although they recognised its presence, it was not a sufficient deterrent to the development of personal relationship. Going beyond the barrier of professional was seen by some as 'a risk', or being 'spontaneous', or 'putting something of oneself in', but nevertheless it was a line that did not limit any of the chaplains interviewed.

It did provide another tension for the chaplains in their offering spiritual care. The rejection of the popular understanding of professionalism—at least the aspect of personal non-involvement—has the potential to create distance between the chaplain and the other team members and is a further challenge associated with the role of the one who is providing spiritual care.

THE EFFICACY OF MINISTRY

In mapping these personal limits to offering spiritual care to those who are dying, the topic of judging the efficacy of one's own ministry was raised and revealed some important concerns. Primarily, there is the acknowledgment of the difficulty in assessing ministry, and a further difficulty that is revealed in the distinction between objective and subjective assessment of efficacy. The former is seen to be a part of the professional ethos, with which the chaplains were not comfortable, a performance-based ethos that has difficulty accessing the reality of relationship and the domain of shared presence. However, the chaplains did not discount objective assessment totally and felt that the comments and supervision of peers was welcome in order to help avoid self-delusion regarding efficacy.

It was generally thought that evidence of realistic assessment is given more by the willingness of patients, families, and staff to trust the chaplain, and to feel free and able to share their concerns. But, fundamentally, most of the chaplains believe that their feelings of belonging and fulfilment are the best criteria for evaluating the efficacy of their ministry. For them, it is whether they believe that they are in the right place, doing the right thing; their feelings of enjoyment, matched by occasional feelings of despair, provide a subjective index to their efficacy. It is one that arises out of their personhood and the relationships that they have formed, not one that has arisen out of institution-based policy.

The question also arises whether the chaplain, with training and expertise in offering spiritual care, has a monopoly within a multidisciplinary team. For example, some nurses might implement chaplain-like strategies but their primary role as a professional healthcarer implies limits to their openness and availability. Similarly, local clergy visiting on request may officiate quite effectively on formal religious occasions, but may lack the sensitivity and understanding to offer spiritual care to those with other faiths or none. The chaplains identified the crucial significance of openness, availability, and sensitivity as essential qualities of spiritual care in the hospice. The value of these qualities in hospice chaplains from the perspective of the patient has been confirmed by Ballard et al. (1999).

FEELINGS AND THE OFFERING OF SPIRITUAL CARE

The importance of feelings in subjective assessment of efficacy cannot be discounted, nor can they be avoided when reflecting on the offering of spiritual care, particularly feelings that might have changed as a consequence of their specific ministry to those who are dying. Many chaplains noted significant changes in feelings, in particular a reduction in fear and anxiety regarding death and dying, and a growth in understanding of the feelings experienced and expressed by those who were dying, feelings such as embarrassment, rejection, alienation, isolation, hurt, and vulnerability.

THE IMAGE OF HUMANKIND

A strong theme running through all the reflections was the image of humanity. This influenced the self-image of the chaplains, how they believed that they were perceived, and their changing perception of humankind. With respect to their self-image, the chaplains noted progressive changes, focusing mainly on a growing appreciation of the gift of life and the relationships that form the essence of their life. There was no evidence of oppressive self-judgment, only acceptance of their humanity, its potential, and a growing awareness of their strengths and weaknesses.

With respect to the image that they believe they project, there was a reluctant acknowledgment of the clerical stereotypes of the 'bumbling fool' or the 'avid evangelist', among others, and the necessity for getting to know the patients in order to dispel these images. The chaplains all expressed the hope that they could come to be seen as a caring friend, or a nonthreatening presence, who might be able to help in some way, if that is what the patient wants.

The overall effect on the chaplains' image of humankind in offering spiritual care to those who are dying was a tendency to become more aware of the compassionate side of human nature, and the uniqueness and value of every human being. One said, '[Being here has] made me aware that there are very few people without a spiritual life. Before, I thought that there were many people who were completely materialistic and now I think that there are very few. And that the divine spark in every human being is more evident than I ever thought it was' (Jenkins 1997, p. 180).

This could be characterised as a Rogerian view, as distinct from the negative Paul–Augustine–Luther view, one that asserts that '… the basic nature of the human being, when functioning freely, is constructive and trustworthy' (Rogers 1961, p. 194). This client-centred perspective corresponds to the belief that the one who is dying should set the agenda of the relationship.

However much these chaplains may have been influenced by psychological theory, their views of relationship, its establishment and limits, their understanding of their ministry, and their perception of self and others, make it clear that they set their offering of spiritual care within a theological understanding.

THE IMAGE OF GOD

It is their theological understanding that helps us to understand most clearly the spiritual caring of these men and women for fellow human beings who are dying. Their understanding of God was not of an all-powerful judge who has to be appeased. Rather, God is the compassionate and caring God, who is revealed in Christ, incarnationally in the compassion and care in human life.

The chaplains clearly believe in this God and in helping to make this divine presence real to those who are dying, those who have an intense need to be accepted and loved. Sometimes it is difficult to feel accepted and loved when even family and friends are rejecting. Christ is seen as a model and the revealer of the presence of the self-giving God. It is this model of self-giving that informs, draws, and supports them as they offer spiritual care to those who are dying.

THE MUTUALITY OF SPIRITUAL CARE

Offering spiritual care involves a mutuality that is often spoken of by chaplains as they make themselves available to the one who is dying. There is something about dying, and being with someone who is dying, that enables a clarity of vision. There is often urgency, an openness, a seeking of intimacy on the part of the patient that is an invitation to those who wish to be present with the other in their experience. So in the relationship between the dying person and the chaplain there is often a mutuality of movement of one towards the other, an opening of selves to each other. Two aspects of this are significant: the power of shared truth, and the relinquishment of self.

The power of shared truth

One of the chaplains described an experience of this mutuality that he labelled 'reciprocal ministry'. He described having experience of this kind of mutuality through being with patients who are

> terminally ill or extremely distressed, in pain, suffering extreme handicap, or suffering from something that makes life for them very hard to bear, they feel that they are completely useless. They feel that they have nothing to give and that the person with them is giving everything and they are receiving; whereas in fact, they are giving out an enormous amount without even knowing it. In fact, I have found that very ill people generate a tremendous spiritual energy and for the most part they are quite unaware of it. When you tell them that they are giving you back something of immense importance, they can't understand what you are saying. But it is tremendously real (Jenkins 1997, p. 123).

This experience of mutuality in the one who is dying meeting the one who is caring is seen in this instance, by this chaplain, as more than simply a meeting of a particular kind. It is understood as a source of nurture, without which he could not imagine his ministry being sustained.

Direct questions about their understanding of death and dying were not put to the chaplains in this study because it focused on their experience of offering spiritual care. However, such understandings, together with the chaplains' understanding of the divine, were interwoven throughout their reflections. More than any other aspect in relation to their ministry, death had come to be recognised as an explicit 'frontier which helps us to see a deeper meaning in life, to refuse to take it for granted, or to trivialise it. A richer quality of life emerges as it is looked at from the perspective of death. To have a proper valuing of life is surely part of what it means to be healed ...' (Wright 1985, p. 70). An important element in this was this truth of the reality of death and its pragmatic expression. There was an honesty revealed by their actions and their striving to make real the love and acceptance of God, to try to help make these real for those fellow human beings who were having to come to terms with the truth of death, in particular perhaps, its 'radical violence'.

In the mutuality of meeting there is also a limit of time, a space between the present and the future, which includes the present, which is filled with possible questions about life past, its meaning, and life present and future. In this context, these are

> intimate questions which call for radical honesty. The honest questions in view of diminishing time can lead into the intimate area where my life comes to its conclusion: 'Indeed, I need no more time. It is good as it is!' In working with the dying one often experiences how the end of life is successfully achieved, and how people after a long period of suffering and, God knows, a painful biography, are able to say and to experience: 'Yes, it is good as it is! I do not need more time.' In this conclusion lies a profound consent to and affirmation of one's life. And in this consent lies a deep realism. It contains knowledge of the openness and brokenness of human life (Viefhues 1996, p. 11).

It is the end of ambition, an end to wanting to be other than we are. It is the acceptance of self and the death of self.

There is, in the meeting, an acknowledgment of the vulnerability of the individual life, but also of the fragility and value of life itself, both of which confront comfort, apathy, and deceit. The power of this mutual understanding lies in its capacity to bring together those who have come to know these fragilities and to provide spiritual nourishment for both of those who are brought together in this knowledge. It is not only consent and affirmation for the one who is dying, but as reciprocal ministry confirms, it is also consent and affirmation for the one who offers the spiritual care, the one who is willing to share the dying intimately.

The honesty that emerges in this domain is quite radical; pretence stands revealed for what it is—empty, and of no value. To pretend that life—or death—is other than it is, in the context of this honesty, is a denial of the particular life that is coming to an end. In being with the person who is dying, sharing the concerns and the dying, to the extent to which this is possible, the chaplain affirms the other and, in return, is affirmed simply by being present, in sharing the consent that is proclaimed in the reality.

In accepting that there is an incompleteness to life, as both must recognise, they are simply drawing a parallel between human life and its history where there is no expectation of perfection, only '… an agreement regarding this broken and ruptured life. "It is good as it is" implies that matters that are unresolved and that remain open are alright as they are' (Viefhues 1996, p. 11). The difference lies in the completeness that is given by death, a completeness that can only exist in history, and this is beyond the personal experience that can be shared with others.

This affirmation extinguishes perfectionism and has a powerful effect on the lives of those who share dying. It is an affirmation of life, an acceptance of the gift and the giver. No one can share the last moments of a life given away without sharing deeply the profound goodness and rightness of death. The power is inestimable because this affirmation

> offers the opportunity to dull one of the sharpest weapons used to oppress the stranger and the self, that is, the weapon that denies me or others dignity. In a culture that draws a wide circle around the weak, the sick and the elderly, this prior creative yes of God to every life, whether it is sick, weak or old, is of the highest importance. God's 'objective' yes to our life is bound to the hope that no life, even if it is broken and worthless in the optic of the individual or collective subjectivity, remains valueless or void of affirmation' (Viefhues 1996, p. 12).

Experiencing such a plenitude of life in the midst of distress has been recognised as an important aspect of the mystery of life and where that happens 'it is always a gift; it can never be forced. A power is revealed there, granting or refusing, which rules in everyday life as much as in extraordinary events' (Pannenberg 1977, p. 40).

Sharing the dying of another is both a part of everyday life and an extra-ordinary event; the power is found in the truth of this and is revealed in mutuality most extensively and intimately.

The relinquishing of self

The sharing of existential truth is not the only dimension of the mutuality of spiritual care. The sharing of self is intrinsically nourishing. Why? In the sharing of dying, it can be seen that there are some who die seemingly focused on themselves, as if they are concentrating all remaining life on itself in order to maintain itself, becoming increasingly withdrawn. Then there is the dying that appears to be shared. In this the dying person is not closed or withdrawn, but increasingly open and giving, as if their dying were a gift to be shared with others.

Letting go, allowing oneself to die, to relinquish the self, is a characteristic of such an awareness in dying. There is no shame, but there is challenge. 'The surrender of self in trusting love to the mystery of the other is the greatest challenge of life ... Our dying, like our living, is fundamentally an act of faith as self-entrustment. It can be a moment of grace' (Sachs 1991, pp. 80–1).

'Letting go' is a common expression in hospice ministry. It is used to describe an act of a dying person, an act that implies that life up to that point has been maintained or held voluntarily, under tension and that finally, when life is released at the will of the one who is dying, that person can then actu-ally die. It is a willed act, a relinquishment of the will to control on the part of the patient. It does not carry the meaning of surrender or defeat, but sig-nifies a knowing deliberation, an acceptance of the inevitable death, and 'precisely my consenting to suffer' (Miller 1988, p. 32).

Nothing can diminish the deep emotional pain and spiritual desolation that can accompany the dying of a parent, child, spouse, or dear friend. Indeed, it is a great contempt for life to romanticise death and dying or to surround it with sentimentality. However, just as we strive for authenticity in life, for authentic living, so it follows that it is possible to strive for authentic dying and to have an understanding of what this might mean.

It seems that an acceptable understanding of being authentic contains an ele-ment of mutuality, in that it means that we accept the unique person we are and, implicitly at least, who the other is, as the basis for our relating. It also means realising the potentialities of life that are peculiarly ours. Authentic dying, there-fore, has about it a sense of freedom from social constraints and expectations.

In those who are dying, a desire for freedom from the superficial and a desire for honesty that transcends material ambition are commonly found. There is generally a desire to be free of the barriers that we place between each other to maintain a safe distance. This is a factor that plays a significant part in the mutuality between the one offering the spiritual care and the one who is dying.

CONCLUSION

Mutuality is given particular prominence in this discussion because it challenges some well-established assumptions about the offering of spiritual care, in particular that the one cared for—the one who is dying—is some kind of passive and helpless recipient of aid. The experience of some of these chaplains makes it possible, however, to think of those who are dying in quite a different light, not as objects of care or as human beings who are empty of value, but as human beings 'who by their very act of dying are prophets speaking to us. Those who feel threatened by death, who hide from it or try to deny it, need the dying and what they can reveal to us of ourselves and of God' (Sachs 1991, p. 81).

It is this belief in the value of each life, in the affirmation of life itself, that empowers these chaplains' offering of spiritual care to those who are dying. If there is a message that they press in any way at all it is that the person who is dying is loved, accepted, and valued, and that therefore their life has fundamental meaning.

REFERENCES

Ballard, P. et al. 1999, 'A perception of hospice chaplaincy', *Contact*, vol. 130, pp. 27–34.

Canetti, E. 1979, *Earwitness*, Seabury Press, London.

Comblin, J. 1990, *Retrieving the Human*, Orbis Books, New York.

Jenkins, W. 1997, 'Caring to death: Reflections on the experience of caring for the dying', unpublished MPhil thesis, Murdoch University, Perth.

Miller, J. A. 1988, *The Way of Suffering: A Geography of Crisis*, Georgetown University Press, Washington, DC.

Pannenberg, W. 1977, *Faith and Reality*, Search Press, London.

Rogers, C. 1961, *On Becoming a Person*, Houghton Mifflin, Boston.

Rumbold, B. D. 1986, *Helplessness and Hope: Pastoral Care in Terminal Illness*, SCM Press, London.

Sachs, J. R. 1991, *The Christian Vision of Humanity*, Liturgical Press, Minnesota.

Viefhues, L. 1996, 'Eternity and the fulfilment of time', *Theology Digest*, vol. 43, no. 1, Spring.

Walter, T. 1997, 'The ideology and organization of spiritual care: Three approaches', *Palliative Medicine*, vol. 11, pp. 21–30.

Wright, F. 1985, *The Pastoral Nature of Healing*, SCM Press, London.

9

Crossing Boundaries

Paul Beirne

The pluralism of contemporary society means that we are aware of difference as never before. In the past cultural boundaries coincided to a significant extent with geographic boundaries, but now, daily life—in most urban areas at least—involves us in encountering, negotiating, or crossing boundaries between different customs, practices, values, and beliefs.

Contemporary approaches to spirituality frequently cross the boundaries between belief systems (Groff 1999). Thus the spiritual quest sometimes leads people to forsake one spiritual–religious tradition for another. Others integrate another tradition into their existing religious or spiritual practice. Some adopt aspects of belief and practice from different traditions, either by drawing intentionally upon a diversity of resources or, less intentionally, by following one of the present-day spiritual writers who themselves draw (frequently without much acknowledgment) on one or more of such spiritual traditions (for example, Myss 1996).

Palliative care has proved to be particularly conducive to the meeting and melding of spiritual traditions. In part this is because palliative care stands in the hospice tradition, which blurred modernism's sharp distinction between the public and private spheres of life (Walter 1994). By insisting that caring for another involves caring about the other, the hospice model of care returned personal spiritual practice and belief to the arena of professional care. In part it is because the imminence of death and the acknowledgment of mortality seem to diminish the importance of many of the distinctions held dear by others in less straitened circumstances. Thus in palliative care we see the boundary between mainstream and complementary therapies blurred or broken down and we see the convergence of religious traditions—in particular

Buddhist belief and practice—brought to bear upon contexts and practices shaped originally by Christian influences (for example, Levine 1987; Singh 1999).

The assertion that we are all spiritual beings, although not necessarily religious beings, implies that any deeply human encounter will have a spiritual dimension. The assertion that each of us expresses our spirituality in unique ways further implies that such deep encounters may challenge and lead to the reshaping of the stories, assumptions, and beliefs that undergird our lives. The challenge of both receiving and offering spiritual care has not been explored to any great extent. In that this challenge is most overt in the encounter between people of different religious persuasions, it may be helpful to explore ways of experiencing and responding to the challenge in these relationships in the hope that this exploration may also shed some light upon constructive ways of meeting the challenge implicit in all mutual encounters.

Boundaries between spiritual traditions may be encountered in various ways: sometimes when a care-giver and a client from different traditions encounter each other, sometimes when a person from one religious tradition chooses to draw on the resources of another, and sometimes through a process of formation in which a care-giver seeks to be formed in more than one tradition or spiritual path. In this chapter, we consider examples of each of these situations and reflect upon some of the implications for the practice of spiritual care in palliative care.

Case study 1—the chaplain

A chaplain at a large metropolitan hospital, who describes himself as a 'traditional, evangelical Presbyterian', shared with me the following experience. Early one morning he was called upon to give the final blessing to a child who had just died. The request came from the child's parents who, he discovered on his way to the child's room, were Chinese Buddhists. 'I was terrified,' he confided to me. 'What was I going to say, or more to the point, what was I going to pray in that room? I know nothing about Buddhism, and nothing in my training prepared me for such a situation. For all I knew, the language that I used would have no meaning and be of less comfort to the poor child's parents.'

He lapsed into silence, recalling the event.

'So what did you do?' I asked, picturing myself in a similar situation.

'Well, I took oils and incense with me, and my Bible, as I suspected that the people, having asked, would expect some reading from our sacred scripture. When I entered the room, the child's parents were standing together beside the bed looking down at their son. They showed no emotion. I nodded to them, lit the incense in a bowl, and placed the bible and the oil on the table. Then I anointed the child and, on the spur of the moment, anointed the parents as well. I was going to read from the bible, but instead something inside me told me to be still. I stood beside the parents, bowed my head, and we remained that way for four or five minutes. Then the child's mother said in a voice just above a whisper:

'Please pray that my child is born into a good family.'

I wondered what my response should be, respecting the wish of the child's parents, yet remaining faithful to my own tradition. After a moment's thought, I prayed that, as Christians believed in a loving and merciful God, their son would, at this moment, be being welcomed into the loving family of the heavenly Father. Then I said farewell to them and their departed son.

'I don't know what effect my words had. The couple remained impassive as I left. It may have been my imagination, but I seem to detect a look of gratitude in the mother's eyes.'

Case study 2—Gene

Gene was a family friend for as long as I can remember. She had emigrated from Malta to Australia in her late teens and married a compatriot, Joseph, soon after her arrival. Gene and Joseph were staunch Catholics. Gene frequently pointed out to us that the Acts of the Apostles recorded that St Paul visited her homeland, and that he had said that 'the inhabitants treated us with unusual kindness' (Acts 28:1). 'We trace our religion back to the very dawn of Christianity,' Gene would tell us with great pride. Gene and Joseph never missed Mass on Sundays and holy days, ate only fish on Friday—even after the ruling was relaxed—and sent their children to Catholic schools. When Joseph died he was buried in the Catholic section of the cemetery after a sung requiem Mass.

Two years ago, Gene contracted cancer, which went into remission for a while but then returned. We, her family and friends, assumed that Gene would take solace in her religion and prepare for death within the parameters of her Catholic faith. She proved us wrong, as least in some respects.

In preparing for death, Gene chose not to spend her last days in a Catholic hospital for the terminally ill. She decided to stay at home. Knowing the strain that would put on her daughter, who would have to look after her, Gene looked for a group to care for her as death approached. She chose Karuna Hospice Service, a Buddhist group that provides free, 24-hour hospice care in the home for people in the last stage of their life. The word 'Karuna' is from the Sanskrit, meaning 'compassion'. Gene was, by all accounts, overwhelmed by the attentive, professional, and loving care of Karuna, who describe themselves as 'volunteers who are simply there, in the home, offering their presence and allowing a situation to unfold in a way that is most helpful.'

These two case studies share some intriguing characteristics and raise several important questions. For example, in the first case, what was the mother of the dead child asking for her son? Did the chaplain understand and respond adequately to her request? In the second case, what would move a traditional Maltese–Australian Roman Catholic to ask a group inspired by Tibetan Mahayana Buddhism to be with her as she approached her final days in this life? Was Gene's decision to request the care of Karuna Hospice Service merely pragmatic, that is, to provide physical aid that could not be provided with regularity and efficiency by another means? Or was there a more spiritual dimension involved? And if there was, what did this group have to offer Gene that helpers in her own tradition lacked?

Without access to the people involved it is not fully possible to answer these questions. However, a response is possible, and I would suggest is necessary, as these cases, far from being isolated, are being replicated in one form or another in hospitals, palliative care services, hospices, and homes all around the country. Chaplains, care workers, and the dying themselves are being faced with new challenges and new opportunities as societies struggle to accept their multicultural and multireligious dimensions.

In the first case, the chaplain envisions eternity spent as part of a loving family in the presence of a benevolent Father. For him, the spirit/soul of the person lying before him has passed on to an eternal state. There is deep sadness in the child's passing, yet equally as deep belief and optimism that what the child is experiencing now is infinitely more desirable than life on earth. It is this message of optimism and consolation that he communicates to the grieving parents.

However, the mother's request to pray that the child is born into a good family indicates a very different attitude to life, death, and what happens to the essence of a person once it passes from the body. To understand her we need to refer to the *Bardo Thödol, The Tibetan Book of the Dead.* In this classic text, the Mahayana Buddhist perspective on the meaning of death and life is explained in graphic detail. The version used here is the third edition of the translation by Dr W. Y. Evans-Wentz (1960), which includes a psychological commentary by Dr Carl Gustav Jung, an introductory foreword by Lama Anagarika Govinda, and a foreword by Sir John Woodroffe. Each of these contributions significantly assists in the understanding of the text.

The *Bardo Thödol*, a book of great antiquity,[1] was first published in English in 1927. In his commentary, Jung describes the book as follows.

> *The Tibetan Book of the Dead*, or the *Bardo Thödol*, is a book of instructions for the dead and dying. Like *The Egyptian Book of the Dead*, it is meant to be a guide for the dead man during the period of his Bardo existence, symbolically described as an intermediate state of forty-nine days' duration between death and rebirth. The text falls into three parts. The first part ... describes the psychic happenings at the moment of death. The second part ... deals with the dream state which supervenes immediately after death, and with what are called 'karmic illusions'. The third part ... concerns the onset of the birth-instinct and of prenatal events. It is characteristic that supreme insight and illumination, and hence the greatest possibility of attaining liberation, are vouchsafed during the actual process of dying. Soon afterward, the 'illusions' begin which lead eventually to reincarnation, the illuminative lights growing ever fainter and more multifarious, and the visions more and more terrifying. This descent illustrates the estrangement of consciousness from the liberating truth as it approaches nearer and nearer to physical rebirth. The purpose of the instruction is to fix the attention of the dead man, at each successive stage of delusion and entanglement, on the ever-present possibility of liberation, and to explain to him the nature of his visions (Evans-Wentz 1960, pp. xxxv–xxxvi).

Obviously, what is described here differs in its very essence from the Christian afterview of death. It should be pointed out, however, that *The*

Tibetan Book of the Dead is not meant to instruct only on what transpires after death or, despite its English title, that this is the book's primary purpose. As Lama Anagarika Govinda points out in the introductory foreword to the book,

> One should not forget that it was originally conceived to serve as a guide not only for the dying and the dead, but for the living as well ... The *Bardo Thödol* is addressed not only to those who see the end of their life approaching, or who are very near death, but to those who still have years of incarnate life before them, and who, for the first time, realize the full meaning of their existence as human beings.
>
> [The] illusoriness of death comes from the identification of the individual with his temporal, transitory form, whether physical, emotional, or mental, whence arise[s] the mistaken notion that there exists a personal, separate egohood of one's own, and the fear of losing it. If, however, the disciple has learned, as the *Bardo Thödol* directs, to identify himself with the Eternal Dharma, the Imperishable Light of Buddhahood within, then the fears of death are dissipated like a cloud before the rising sun. Then he knows that whatever he may see, hear, or feel, in the hour of his departure from this life, is but a reflection of his own conscious and subconscious mental content; and no mind-created illusion can then have power over him if he knows its origin and is able to recognize it. The illusory Bardo visions vary, in keeping with the religious or cultural tradition in which the percipient has grown up, but their underlying motive-power is the same in all human beings. Thus it is that the profound psychology set forth by the *Bardo Thödol* constitutes an important contribution to our knowledge of the human mind and of the path that leads beyond it. Under the guise of a science of death, the *Bardo Thödol* reveals the secret of life; and therein lies its spiritual value and its universal appeal (Evans-Wentz 1960, pp. lxi–lxiii).

We might be tempted at this point to enter into an examination of the fundamental Buddhist concepts that occur in the above quotations, such as 'illusoriness of death', 'karmic illusions', 'the Eternal Dharma, the Imperishable Light of Buddhahood within'. This would not only be a distraction, but would also entail a philosophical and semantic examination of such complexity that the focus of this chapter would be lost. What can be gleaned from these quotations is that there is a profound difference between Christian and Buddhist approaches to death, not to mention the meaning and purpose of life. Sir John Woodroffe outlines this difference as follows.

> The doctrine of 'Reincarnation' on the one hand and of 'Resurrection' on the other is the chief difference between the four leading Religions—Brahmanism,

Buddhism, Christianity, and Islam. Christianity, in its orthodox form, rejects the most ancient and widespread belief of the *Kúklos genesean*, or *Sangsara*, or 'Reincarnation', and admits one universe only—this, the first and last—and two lives, one here in the natural body and one hereafter in the body of Resurrection … The latter doctrine limits man's lives to two in number, of which the first or present determines for ever the character of the second or future.

Brahmanism and Buddhism would accept the doctrine that 'as a tree falls so shall it lie', but they deny that it so lies forever. To the adherents of these two kindred beliefs this present universe is not the first and last. It is but one of an infinite series, without absolute beginning or end, though each series of the universe appears and disappears. They also teach a series of successive existences therein until morality, devotion, and knowledge produce that high form of detachment which is the cause of Liberation from the cycle of birth and death called 'The Wandering' (or *Sangsara*). Freedom is the attainment of the Supreme State called the Void, Nirvana, and by other names (Evans-Wentz 1960, p. lxvii)

From the request of the mother of the dead child it can be deduced that she believed her son to be continuing on his *Sangsara*, wandering, existence, and her wish for him, naturally, was that his next birth be a progression on his last. How would this progression be achieved? In other words, what is the process, from a Buddhist point of view, through which a deceased person is reborn into new life?

According to the *Bardo Thödol*, the deceased is faced with two options immediately after death, specifically between Sangsara and Nirvana. The latter term is a this-worldly and thus inadequate description of the release from birth, death, and their pains. This state is also described as the 'Perfect Experience which is Buddahood', or 'Consciousness freed of all limitation'; it is a 'timeless state' which, from the emotional aspect, is 'pure Bliss unaffected by sorrow' and from a volitional aspect, is 'freedom of action and almighty power (Evans-Wentz 1960, p. lxxii). It is a state arrived at only by adepts who have achieved enlightenment through faithfulness to the Four Noble Truths. These Truths are as follows.

1 There is suffering.
2 Suffering is caused.
3 Suffering can be extinguished by eliminating the causes of suffering.
4 The way to extinguish the cause of suffering is to follow the Middle Way of the Noble Eightfold Path[2] (Koller 1985, pp. 136–7, 140–1).

The vast majority of individuals, however, do not progress to this timeless state but continue on in the Sangsara state, wandering through the worlds of birth and death. The *Bardo Thödol* could be described as a traveller's guide to these worlds, in particular the world a person encounters between death and rebirth. To the grieving parents, the consciousness of their child was travelling through this intermediary state as they stood beside his inert body.

The *Bardo Thödol* describes the stages of the journey between death and rebirth as follows. At the point of death the deceased—if he or she does not realise the Void and become a Buddha but continues on the life of the flesh—must experience the 'Six Worlds, or *Lokas* ('that which is experienced', Evans-Wentz 1960, p. lxxii). Lokas are apparitions that veil the mind from the Clear Light of the Void. The apparitions stem from what are referred to as the 'Six Poisons'—pride, jealousy, sloth, anger, greed, lust—which bear a remarkable resemblance to the seven deadly sins of Christianity.[3]

The *Bardo*[4] period lasts for forty-nine days and consists of three states. The first Bardo state, the *Chikhai Bardo*, or 'Transitional State of the Moment of Death', lasts for approximately four days. During this state, the Knower, or principle of consciousness, in the case of an ordinary person, is in a trance-like state and is unaware that it has been separated from the human-plane body. During this state, the Clear Light mentioned above dawns, but the ordinary person is only able to perceive it in an obscured way and is unable to remain in the transcendental state and passes on to the second state of *Chönyid Bardo*. It is in this state that there dawns on the person in transition the hallucinations mentioned above which are created by the karmic actions done by him or her during a previous life (Evans-Wentz 1960, pp. 28–9). Evans-Wentz comments that,

> In the Second *Bardo*, the deceased is, unless otherwise enlightened, more or less under the delusion that although he is deceased he still possesses a body like the body of flesh and blood. When he comes to realize that really he has no such body, he begins to develop an overmastering desire to possess one; and seeking for one, the karmic predilection enters into the Third *Bardo* of seeking Rebirth, and eventually, with his rebirth in this or some other world, the after-death state comes to an end.
>
> The Third *Bardo* is called the *Sidpa Bardo* (Transitional State of [or while seeking] Rebirth), which ends when the principle of consciousness has taken rebirth in the human or some other world, or in one of the paradise realms (Evans-Wentz 1960, pp. 29–30).

Rebirth as a human being is of utmost importance, as this is the only hope for the ordinary person of ultimately reaching Buddhahood. As Evans-Wentz points out, rebirth in any other than the human world delays the reaching of this final goal (1960, p. 30).

This, then, is at the heart of the mother's request for her deceased son, that he would pass safely through the three *Bardo* levels and be reborn into a good family. Her grief is mixed with a continuing passionate and maternal interest in the individual whose cycles of lives intersected with hers all too briefly. Her one-sentence request reveals an ongoing love and concern for her son. It also reveals a system of belief that differs in almost all its aspects from that of the chaplain who stood at her side.

This difference comes into sharp relief if we consider exactly what the *Bardo* stipulates about life, death, and the stages in between. Specifically, heavens, hells, and other worlds are entirely dependent on phenomena that are illusionary and unreal, except in the Sangsaric mind perceiving them. Gods, demons, or spirits do not exist. They are merely imaginings and are dependent on a cause, namely, the thirsting after sensation. Until this cause is overcome by Enlightenment, death follows birth, and birth death, unceasingly. The afterdeath experience is merely a continuation, under altered conditions, of the existence in the human world; the nature of the existence between death and rebirth is determined by antecedent actions. The afterdeath experience is a prolonged dream-like state filled with hallucinatory visions directly resultant on the mental content of the percipient, that is, the visions will be happy and heaven-like if the *karma* (actions, effect of actions) of the percipient is good; the visions will be miserable and hell-like if the *karma* is bad (Evans-Wentz 1960, pp. 66–7).

The ultimate goal of Buddhism, as reaffirmed by the *Bardo Thödol*, is not to spend eternal life in the company of a benevolent deity and other fortunate souls as envisioned by adherents of Christian denominations, but is, rather, to achieve Enlightenment through realising the unreality of existence and experiencing Nirvana.[5] Simply put, unlike Christianity, which teaches dependence upon an outside power or saviour, Buddhism teaches dependence on self-exertion alone in the gaining of salvation (Evans-Wentz 1960, p. 235).

How, then, does a spiritual care or a palliative care worker operating out of a particular belief or ethical system respond adequately to a person with radically different world and afterworld perspectives? The example here contrasts Buddhist and Christian beliefs. Yet this is merely a metaphor for the extraordinary cultural and religious diversity that spiritual and palliative care workers are faced with on a daily basis in a multicultural, multireligious society. Is a meeting of minds and hearts possible? Or are belief systems so intrinsically and radically different that they preclude any empathetic interaction?

The two case studies at the beginning of this chapter suggest a negative response to this latter question. Even though, by his own admission, the chaplain knew very little about the belief system of the grieving couple, he nevertheless responded with sensitivity and compassion to the parents' loss. Perhaps they sensed that he was responding to them and to their pain as well as to his own calling, and his compassion (a virtue at the very centre of Buddhist belief and practice) communicated more than any word or symbol could possibly do. It is little wonder that the mother expressed her appreciation in a thoroughly cultural way: not with words or gestures, but with a look of gratitude in her eyes.

It may have been this virtue of compassion—among others—that drew Gene to engage the services of Karuna Hospice Service in the last days of her life. The organisation is described thus: 'Inspired by Tibetan Buddhist philosophies and based on the principles of love, compassion and respect of life, Karuna offers free care 24 hours a day, seven days a week. It enables those with a life-threatening illness to die at home with peace and dignity, and supports the physical, emotional, intellectual and spiritual needs of the dying person, their family and friends' (National Community Link 1999).

If one substituted the word 'Christian', or any other religious tradition for that matter, for 'Tibetan Buddhist' in the above description, it would not seem out of place. Naturally, one must be cautious in implying a reductionism that renders meaningless the uniqueness and diversity of the faith and ethical structures of each religious tradition. Yet there is a communality evident here that becomes apparent as individuals face the most fundamental questions of their existence. I suggest that it is at this point that the spiritual realm takes precedence over the religious. In other words, an individual who is facing imminent death becomes more interested in the very substance of life rather than its rituals and that, at this point, spirituality takes precedence over dogma. An organisation that is based on the principles of love, compassion, and respect for life and that enables those with a life-threatening illness to die at home with peace and dignity, regardless of whether it originates in the religion one professes to live by, must appear worthy of consideration in one's final days. Gene certainly thought so.

I would hazard a guess that Gene was totally unfamiliar with the *Bardo Thödol* and, if asked, would have been hard pressed to identify even one of the Four Noble Truths or the Noble Eightfold Path. Yet by all accounts she deeply appreciated the love and compassion she received from the volunteers of Karuna. One could say that she was eternally grateful to them.

In one's final days, peace and harmony are life-sustaining values. They offer essential sustenance to the spirit as the body weakens. The dying have little truck with divisions and distinctions. It is at the point of death that that which is at the heart of all religions becomes immediate and is, in a fundamental way, indistinguishable.

A feature of today's multicultural societies is the growing number of people choosing to practice more than one religious tradition (Gilmour 2000). In the latter half of a sixteen-year sojourn in South Korea I had the opportunity to study and experience at first hand Tonghak, the country's first New Religious Movement. Perhaps the term 'New' is slightly misleading, as Tonghak, founded in 1860, is approaching its one hundred and fiftieth anniversary. During this time the religion has undergone significant changes, even to the extent of changing its name from Tonghak (Eastern Learning) to Ch'ondo-gyo (Religion of the Heavenly Way). Yet its fundamental principles remain the same as when it was first promulgated.

I first heard of the founder of the religion, Ch'oe Che-u, in a Korean history class. Something about Ch'oe's life and early death made a deep impression, and I found myself being drawn deeper and deeper into his story. Eventually, I spent years writing a PhD dissertation on Ch'oe's religious experience and assisted in translating his scriptures into English (Beirne 1999). These were by no means purely academic exercises. In Ch'oe I found a religious mentor and guide who challenged and eventually affirmed the very core of my own beliefs. In his eclectic and egalitarian creed I discovered a wisdom and a wellspring that caused me to reflect on the uniqueness and universality of all religions.

Ch'oe's birth as the son of a disenfranchised nobleman and his third wife branded him a *soja*, one of a floating, dispossessed subgroup who could expect to play no effective role in a strict hierarchical society that barely recognised their existence. Despite showing an early brilliance and being classically trained by his father in the neo-Confucian tradition, because of his lack of status Ch'oe could not sit for government examinations; he was forced to travel around the country selling wares to support his increasingly impoverished family.

During his years of wandering, Ch'oe experienced a land in chaos. Moved by the fear and suffering of his people, Ch'oe decided that a spiritual renaissance was the answer to his country's internal and external problems. Viewing the old religions as being too antiquated and exhausted to cope with the crisis at hand and their leaders too obsessed with theoretical arguments that had no relevance to the situation of the general populace, Ch'oe acted. Retiring with his family to a retreat his father built in the Kumi mountain range overlooking the ancient Silla capital of Kyongju, Ch'oe meditated for lengthy periods until, on 5 April 1860, he underwent an epiphany in which, by his own account, the infinite Great Way of Truth was revealed to him by Hanul-Nim, the Lord of Heaven.

As a result of this experience, Ch'oe promulgated his new religious creed by using two potent symbols, which he created from classic sources and folk religion. The first was the Yongbu, a sacred talisman that believers wrote on a piece of white paper with Zenlike concentration, then burnt the paper and consumed it with pure water. The physical healing that took place as a result of this ritual was an external manifestation of an inner union with the divine. The second symbol was a twenty-one Chinese character chant, a doctrinal statement that described the spiritual relationship between the devotee and the Lord of Heaven. This chant was performative in that it achieved what its words expressed, specifically, unity with the most powerful spiritual force in the universe. The two symbols were complementary, one stressing an individual act of union (Yongbu), the other a communal act (Chumun).

With these two symbols as the centrepiece of his religion, Ch'oe wrote two books of scripture, one in Chinese characters and one in Korean, in traditional Kasa verse. The core of Ch'oe's message was that all people, regardless of status, gender, intellectual capability, or age, had the Lord of Heaven residing in their hearts and could access this most powerful Being through proper use of the Yongbu and Chumun. He taught that all divisions in society were merely human inventions which separated rather than united and were thus fundamentally flawed. Ch'oe's radical egalitarianism was supported by a seminal statement in his scriptures, spoken by the Lord of Heaven to Ch'oe during his epiphany. Hanul-Nim said, 'My heart is your heart. But how could humanity know this?' (Cho'oe Che-u 1983).

Ch'oe believed that he was chosen by the Lord of Heaven to disseminate this truth, that it was possible for a human to be so united with the divine, that their hearts were identical. According to the Korea scholar John Duncan, this identification of human with the divine implied 'a fundamental equality of all human beings not to be found in either the Chinese or the indigenous heritage' (1996, p. 314).

Ch'oe's promulgation of his religion lasted for little over three years. Branded as a subversive because his teachings challenged the fundamental precepts of neo-Confucianism, Ch'oe was arrested, tried, and sentenced to death. Immediately prior to the sentence being carried out, Ch'oe asked his jailer for a bowl of pure water. The request granted, he placed the bowl beside him, prayed quietly, and faced death peacefully in the belief that, having attained union with the most powerful force in the universe, he had nothing to fear from earthly authorities whose power was rooted in their own transient mortality.

Following Ch'oe's death all his writings were burnt; his followers were forced to flee to the mountains. Yet Ch'oe's teachings had lit a spark in the hearts of a populace who had long since lost faith in the official ethic of the ruling classes. His scriptures were rewritten from memory by the second leader of the Tonghaks and his religious teachings spread like wildfire. His principles of 'All Life Evolves Toward Social Unity', 'The Kingdom of Heaven on Earth', and 'Bearing the Lord of Heaven Within' inspired a dispirited populace to address the corruption that pervaded the nation. A militant arm of the movement instigated the Tonghak peasant revolution in 1894, the suppression of which by Japanese troops aiding inferior government forces led to the outbreak of the Sino-Japanese war. The Japanese victory in this conflict began of one of the darkest periods in Korean history, the humiliating and oppressive occupation of the country by Japan. During this thirty-five-year occupation, a passive yet dynamic resistance movement spread across the country, out of which evolved a Declaration of Korean Independence promulgated on 1 March 1919. Its chief signatory was Son Pyong-hi, the third leader of the Tonghak/Ch'ondo-gyo religion. Sixteen of the thirty-three national leaders who signed the document were Tonghak/Ch'ondo-gyo members.

Ch'oe Che-u's life and death proved again how much easier it is to kill the prophet than to kill his dream.

My journey through Ch'oe's life and its aftermath was inspiring and instructive on many levels. Just one of these I will address now. I had the honour of translating Ch'oe's scriptures into English with a small team of scholars led by Ch'oe Chong-dae, a direct descendant of Ch'oe Si-hyong, the second leader of the Tonghaks, the man responsible for guiding the religion through its most difficult period following the death of its founder. In grappling with the complexities of translating East Asian thinking and principles into language comprehensible to a Western mind, I came to know and admire Ch'oe

Chong-dae and spent many pleasant hours with him, his wife, and their two young sons. It came as a great shock when, after a short illness, Mr Ch'oe's wife died, leaving him to raise his four- and seven-year-old boys.

I attended the funeral with deep sadness and a total inability to address in even the most rudimentary way my friend's profound loss. According to Korean practice, I visited the funeral parlour, removed my shoes, lit an incense stick, bowed my head before the picture of the deceased, and said a silent prayer. I then turned to Mr Ch'oe and his family, bowed, and was struck speechless. Aware of my distress, Mr Ch'oe took me by the arm, led me outside, and spoke to me quietly. It occurred to me then that it was he who was doing the consoling.

Reflecting later on his calmness and his compassion, I could not but recall the words that the Lord of Heaven spoke to Ch'oe Che-u at his father's retreat on Mt Kumi: 'My heart is your heart. But how could humanity know this?'

If one believes that not only one's own heart but those of one's companions are in complete union with the universal source of power and wisdom, then life and death take on a completely different meaning. With my Western mentality and Judaeo-Christian upbringing, I am still not conversant with this meaning. Yet I remember clearly a gentle woman who did believe this way and who faced life and death with courage, dignity, and hope. And I remember a gentle man who comforted me in the midst of his own grief and who guided me to understand and embrace the foreign until it became familiar.

Before I left Korea, I made a pilgrimage to the Dragon Pool Pavilion on Mt Kumi where Ch'oe Che-u underwent his ecstatic encounter with the Lord of Heaven. Unlike the hacking pollution in the megalopolis from which I had just journeyed, the mountain air was crisp and clean, and vibrant colours danced off leaves and flowers. A tumbling stream bubbled over rocks just outside the pagoda-shaped Pavilion, and birds and cicadas sang in the thick forest that surrounded it. I entered the Pavilion and sat directly in front of an artist's rendition of Ch'oe Che-u, on the spot where he reputedly conversed with his Lord.

I closed my eyes and chanted the twenty-one Chinese character chant. Then, following Ch'oe's instructions, I emptied my mind, quieted my heart, and tried to be still.

I have no idea how long I sat there. The sun had set behind the hills when I left. The birds and cicadas were silent. But my heart was singing.

❖

In the examples given above, the crossing—or transcending—of boundaries takes place at points of genuine human encounter, in relationships in which people are open and vulnerable to each other, and where each treats the other with due honour and respect. In such encounters all systems of belief seem to be preliminary to an actual experience that opens us up to possibility and transformation. In this respect at least some of the contemporary popular writers on spirituality seem to be right: it is spiritual practice rather than the mastery of particular systems of belief that should receive highest priority.

The process of spiritual maturing that allows us to live and to die to the fullness of our abilities is indicated in the Ten Oxherding Pictures, an ancient Taoist meditative practice that has been adopted by Zen Buddhism. It is a pictorial representation of an individual's quest for enlightenment. In the pictures, the ox symbolises the Ultimate, undivided reality (the Buddha nature), which is the ground of all existence. The oxherd is the self who, because of its individuated ego, is separated from the ox, but with progressive enlightenment comes to realise its fundamental identity in the ultimate reality that transcends all distinctions. When this happens, the oxherd self realises the ultimacy of all existence as well as the preciousness and profundity of the most ordinary things in life, and thereby illuminates all creation with this enlightenment (Koller 1985, pp. 224–5).

The pictures can be summarised as follows:

the first picture shows the oxherd searching for his lost ox. In the second picture he finds the tracks of the ox, bringing hope that his ox is not lost forever. In the third picture he catches sight of the ox. The fourth picture shows the oxherd catching the ox, using a bridle to control it. (This picture symbolises the discipline required of the Zen practitioner.) The fifth picture, in which the ox willingly follows the oxherd home, illustrates that this discipline brings the practitioner into accord with the true nature of reality. The sixth picture represents the tranquillity and harmony that reunion with the source of existence brings; the oxherd rides on the back of the ox, joyously playing his flute. In the seventh picture the oxherd becomes one with the ox; it is no longer necessary to represent the ox pictorially, for it is none other than the true self. The eighth picture, of an empty circle, indicates that, when the duality of the self has been overcome, not only is reality (the ox) forgotten but so also is the self (the oxherd); the circle symbolises the all-encompassing emptiness that constitutes the ground of all being. The ninth picture illustrates that when self and reality are left behind, things are revealed to be just as they are; streams flow on of themselves, and flowers and trees bloom naturally in vibrant colours. In the tenth picture, the oxherd enters the marketplace, doing everyday, ordinary things. He immerses himself in the world, sharing his enlightened existence with all around him, leading all those he encounters in the way of Buddha. And, through the radiance of his life, he brings withered trees to bloom (Koller 1985, p. 151).

The reason for mentioning the Ten Oxherding Pictures is threefold. First, an explanation of the symbolic representation that is at the heart of Zen Buddhist practice may foster an understanding of the religion itself and the Mahayana Buddhist goal of becoming a *Bodhisattva*, the enlightened individual described in Pictures eight through ten, the *Bodhisattva* being a person whose only concern is to help others extinguish their suffering.[6] It is an ideal that the volunteers of Karuna Hospice Service seek to realise.

Second, the pictures can also represent, by association, the struggle individuals can enter into when coming to terms with their own mortality. In other words, the Pictures can represent the quest for the true self that becomes most immediate in the face of death.

Third, the Pictures can also represent the struggle and the triumph in the life and in the death of Ch'oe Che-u and the blossoming that followed in the lives and in the deaths of his followers. The expression of struggle and triumph in Tonghak/Ch'ondo-gyo, Buddhism, and other religions are expressed in their particular rituals and symbols. But it would be a tragedy if the particularity of these symbols and rituals could not be appreciated and treasured universally by all religious traditions.

Perhaps the harmony expressed in nonsequential Pictures eight through ten can occur naturally in the final moments of life. Certainly the imminence of death can bring to the fore the search for mystical experience that underlies, and is the foundation of, religious belief systems (Teasdale 1999) and of human spirituality in all its diversity and depth.

REFERENCES

Beirne, P. L. 1999, 'The eclectic mysticism of Ch'oe Che-u', *Review of Korean Studies*, vol. 2, pp. 159–82.

Ch'oe Che-u 1983, 'Nonhak-mun [Discussion on Truth] Tonggyong Taechon [Great Collection of Eastern Scriptures]', *Chondo-gyo Kyongchon* [*Ch'ondo-gyo Scriptures*], Ch'ondo-gyo Central Headquarters, Seoul.

Duncan, J. 1996, 'The emergence of the Tonghak religion', *Sourcebook of Korean Civilization*, in P. Lee (ed.), Columbia University Press, New York, pp. 313–16.

Evans-Wentz, W. Y. (trans.) 1960, *The Tibetan Book of the Dead*, 3rd edn, Oxford University Press, Oxford.

Gilmour, P. 2000, 'Spiritual borderlands: Practising more than a single religious tradition', *Listening: Journal of Religion and Culture*, vol. 35, no. 1, pp. 17–24.

Groff, L. 1999, 'Crossing boundaries: Spiritual journeys in search of the sacred', *Concilium*, no. 2, pp. 116–24.

Koller, J. M. 1985, *Oriental Philosophies*, 2nd edn, Scribner, New York.

Levine, S. 1987, *Healing into Life and Death*, Anchor, New York.

Myss, C. 1996, *Anatomy of the Spirit*, Bantam Books, Sydney.

National Community Link 1999, Issue 11, December.

Singh, K. D. 1999, *The Grace in Dying*, Newleaf, Dublin.

Teasdale, W. 1999, 'Mysticism as the crossing of ultimate boundaries', *Concilium*, no. 2, pp. 90–4.

Walter, T. 1994, *The Revival of Death*, Routledge, London.

NOTES

1   Evans-Wentz notes that the *Bardo Thödol* text was first committed to writing in the eighth century AD.

2   The Noble Eightfold Path and the qualities that exemplify each aspect are:

1 Right views	
2 Right resolution	Wisdom
3 Right speech	
4 Right action	
5 Right livelihood	Conduct
6 Right effort	
7 Mindfulness	Mental Discipline
8 Right concentration	

3   Woodroffe (Evans-Wentz 1960, p. lxxiii) notes that the Hindus call these the Six Enemies.

4   *Bar-do* literally means 'between two', that is, between two states—death and rebirth (Evans-Wentz 1960, p. 28).

5   Although defying conventional definition, *Nirvana* can be regarded in simple if simplistic terms as an unconditioned and nontransitory state of sufferingless existence. The Buddha Gautama speaks of it thus: 'There is, disciples, a Realm devoid of

earth and water, fire and air. It is not endless space, not infinite thought, nor nothingness, neither ideas nor non-ideas. Not this world nor that is it. I call it neither a coming nor a departing, nor a standing still, nor death, nor birth; it is without a basis, progress, or a stay; it is the ending of sorrow.' (*Ud na*, viii. 1, 4, 3; based on a translation from the original *Pali* by Francis J. Payne, and quoted in Evans-Wentz 1960, p. 68).

6   It should be noted that the pictures are sequential up to and including number seven, but eight, nine, and ten are expressions of the same reality.

10

Supervision and Spirituality for the Care-givers

John E. Paver

I write from three perspectives: as a pastor with thirteen years experience in caring for people with cancer, as a pastoral supervisor who has supervised students who have cared for people with cancer, and as a person who has been diagnosed with an aggressive prostate cancer. I am pastor, educator, and patient.[1] I am writing here about the supervision of care-givers as it relates to their spirituality. It could be imagined that my threefold involvement might blur the boundaries and restrict my ability to write on this subject but, on the contrary, it has enriched my understanding of what it means not only to care for myself but also to care for others. Each aspect of involvement has given me a different angle on what it means to offer spiritual care to people with cancer and supervision to people who are caring for people with cancer. Much of what I write stems from my own experience of cancer. In fact, it might be classified as self-supervision as I struggle to integrate the personal, pastoral, and faith issues of my life. My intention in this chapter is to define an understanding of integration as it relates to spirituality and from there to address the factors that undermine spirituality, then, finally, develop some supervisory responses to these issues.

One of the suspects in two murders committed in Elizabeth George's recent novel, *In Pursuit of the Proper Sinner* (1999), is Andy Maiden, formerly a police officer in an elite undercover unit. His duties as an undercover agent required him to take on a succession of false identities and acts that are contrary to his character. Since his retirement he has been in ill health, both emotionally and physically. His wife Nan has not been able to get an accurate diagnosis from the many doctors Andy has visited. Eventually, one offers not a diagnosis but an explanation.

Unfortunately, considering the type of work he does, your husband can't live a dichotomous life; she was told after months and years of visiting doctors. Not, that is, if he wishes to be completely integrated as an individual ... Andrew can't live a life of contradictions, Mrs Maiden. He can't compartmentalise. He can't assume an identity at odds with his central persona. It's the adoption of a succession of identities that appears to be causing this failure of part of his nervous system (George 1999, pp. 393–4).[2]

THE ISSUE OF INTEGRATION

These words strike at the core of people who have been diagnosed with cancer. To be so diagnosed and to face the possibility of death tests the credibility of the life you have led. It is my belief that people who have led a congruent and integrated life (no matter the details of their beliefs) will be able to face their cancer and live courageously and creatively until their death. I have observed this in others, and I hope it is eventually a reality for myself. It has also been my observation that people who assume an identity at odds with their central character or lead dichotomous lives are less likely to face their cancer in ways that will be enriching to them. I do not intend a moral judgment on such people, but I do stand by the statement 'You die the way you live'. Further, people who care for people with cancer, if they care deeply, will also face many of the same issues with which the person with cancer is confronted. These issues may appear in the subtexts of people's lives and be identified, for instance, as the fear of incompleteness, the dread of abandonment, or the terror of losing control. The confrontation can make or break many carers, and it is in this encounter that supervision seeks to give assistance.

During my early months as chaplain at the Peter MacCallum Cancer Institute in Melbourne I was unable to recognise that many of the issues I encountered in patients were also mine, and this led to a personal and professional crisis. I am sure the patients were aware of my incongruence and could see through my pretence. In this wonderful institution pastoral integrity and honesty were called for; self-deception was not tolerated. It was only as I owned my fear and let go of my control that I experienced new life, which enabled me to enter people's lives and provide some hope through my understanding of the Gospel.

Integration and spirituality

George does not specifically refer to spirituality when she uses the words 'integration' and 'central persona' in her novel. It is, however, my contention that integration is at the heart of spirituality, especially in the raw experience of the person with cancer and, sometimes, the carer. Cancer will not allow us to separate the body and the spirit. Nelson Thayer (1985) believes that the metaphor 'integration' is significant for spirituality as it suggests a progressive coherence and deeper ranges of experience and reality in the being and identity of the person. He gives attention to the private and corporate disciplines that Christians through the centuries have found conducive to a relationship with the mystery of God. He continues: 'But these disciplines ... will all share one fundamental quality: they carry the person into, not away from, lived experience. So much is this the case that awareness of transcendence may in fact be indistinguishable from the awareness of immanence ... Disciplines of prayer, worship, and engagement with the world are vehicles for the awareness of God present in, permeating, emerging from our lived experience' (Thayer 1985, p. 57). For Thayer, mind and body, intellect and feeling, belief and action are not in opposition: they are complementary modes of experiencing and responding to what is. People with cancer may not formally understand this conception of spirituality, but in most cases there is a very strong connection between what is happening to them as people and what is happening to their souls. People search for answers and in doing so are searching for meaning for their lives. For me, how a person integrates lived experience is the ongoing quest for spiritual formation.

There is no set prescription for everyone. Integration is to be understood as a journey, a process, not as a prescribed state. This is why images of movement, not attainment, are appropriate for spirituality. Thayer suggests that ' "Journey", "pilgrimage", "spinning", and "weaving"—at times "wandering"—these are the metaphors of Christian spiritual formation' (Thayer 1985, p. 60). For this reason we need to journey until the day we die. I am aware that for many people with cancer, and their carers, this understanding of spirituality could be threatening because it does not have the permanency that many require for a crisis. I do understand that for some people their security is based on the belief that their faith is unchanging and that God remains the same, and during a crisis this belief gives meaning. But I have witnessed the viciousness of the cancer that eats into people's souls or unchanging faith, leaving them helpless and hopeless.

If spirituality has to do with making connections between the human and the divine, then supervision takes on the responsibility of assisting the carer in making these connections. As a supervisor I see my role as being that of both a role model and an educator who challenges, supports, intervenes, and assists in pursuit of a vision that allows these connections to be made. However, as with most connections, there are also tensions, and there are three in particular upon which I wish to concentrate. They are:

- the tension between remembering and forgetting
- the tension between closeness and distance
- the tension between caring about and receiving care.

The tension between remembering and forgetting

My four-year-old grandson and I often visit the Melbourne General Cemetery. Many of the graves are well preserved; others, which are very old and neglected, with the brickwork cracking and crumbling, lead to some vivid, imaginative excursions. My grandson enjoys going and asks many questions, some of which I struggle to answer, at least to provide an answer which makes sense to him, let alone me. I have tried to teach him to respect the sanctity of life and death during our visits. Recently, my five-year-old grandson joined us on a visit. An outgoing and gregarious boy, he is not shy in expressing his opinions. He was fascinated by the 'trophies' (flower urns) and the statues of Jesus, Mary, the baby Jesus, and the angels that protected many of the graves. At one point he demanded that we all stand in an attitude of prayer before a statue of the adult Jesus and offer our prayers to him. It was a moving and poignant moment as my younger grandson and I stood with him, our hands in a position of prayer, looking at the image of Jesus. A discussion on a number of topics followed, which included the age of gravesites and why some were attended while others were neglected. We talked about the ages of family members and those who were old and those who were young. I appreciated the respect, naturalness, and spontaneity in my grandsons when they asked life and death questions at a level that touched me.

In many ways I was touched too by the symbolism of the attended and neglected gravesites. My terminal cancer confronts me with the questions: Who will remember me and who will forget me? For what will I be remembered? I know I will be remembered; but for how long? I hope that I will not be forgotten too quickly. My underlying belief is that I will live on when I am not forgotten. This view might seem egotistical, but it is consistent with the biblical view, which commands us to remember (1 Corinthians 11:23–6). It would not be sacrilegious to suggest that part of new life embraces remembering.

My cancer has reminded me of some things I had forgotten. I am sure that they have been in the background but the cancer brings them into my consciousness. Some of them need attending to. Perhaps most important is the question whether I have a life that is authentic and genuine, one that can sustain me in the reality of the possibility of death. The most significant theme in my life has been my striving for unity of life and thought. I have endeavoured to live an authentic and integrated life. It has been the basis for my personhood, ministry, and faith. Intrinsic to this belief is the premise that memory is vital and gives meaning to human life. It is my contention that some memories (events and engagements) not dealt with, suppressed, not incorporated into one's being, can have a detrimental effect on one's personhood, spirituality, and ministry. To forget these important events for whatever reason can have far-reaching implications, as Freud, for one, reminded us (Freud 1917).[3] The impact of this nonengagement with significant events can produce a life of self-deception. For instance, nonengagement is often located in unresolved grief. For many, the grief experience is too painful to engage, or could became too disruptive to their present understanding of selfhood; therefore, the spelling out of this engagement is habitually avoided. It is the nonincorporation or lack of integration of significant events into our lives that can lead to tragic circumstances when we are faced with the ultimate threat of death. It takes courage to face our avoidances or disengagements and it takes some skill by the carer to assist people to do so.

For me, the greatest threat to this desire for integration comes from a narrative outside myself that threatens to fragment my striving for authenticity. This threat to my spirituality is the hormone treatment I receive for the purpose of containing my cancer. The ingredients of this treatment have their own narratives, which impose themselves on mine. So far the treatment has contained the cancer, but its impact on me has been so deleterious that I have suspended it. The treatment makes me something other than I am. It not only makes me physically ill, but it also challenges my inner being. I am thankful for the extension of my lifespan through this treatment, but its aggressiveness and spirit-changing potential cannot go unchallenged. In fact, most of our conventional treatments for cancer have aggressive narratives with militaristic overtones. For instance, radiotherapy uses penetrating rays to kill the tumour, chemotherapy invades the whole body system to attack cancer cells, surgery is an excision of the tumour, immunology involves fighting fire with fire, while hormone treatment places a foreign substance into the body to reduce the level of testosterone that feeds the cancer. These conventional forms of treatment are symbols of masculine power and strength. We need these symbols, but my concern is for vulnerable people and the people of peace. The impact of these treatments with their aggressive symbolism has the potential to erode our spirit and being.

Up to this point I have been writing as a patient. I will now adopt my supervisory role and discuss the implications of remembering and forgetting for those who care for people with cancer. It is a well-known aphorism that our patients or our students are our best teachers and, if we take the saying seriously, we cannot help but address the issues which our patients or students are facing. I have written elsewhere of the importance of memory in the development of personhood and spirituality (Paver 1994). As supervisor and educator I endeavour to address the importance of remembering in two ways: first, through autobiography, and second, through verbatim writing.

TOOLS FOR SUPERVISION

Autobiographical writing

The importance of memory in my clinical pastoral education practice is signalled by the autobiography that each student is expected to write as part of the application form for acceptance into the program. In their autobiography applicants are expected to locate significant events that have been turning points in their lives. Such events may be a religious experience, the loss of a loved one through divorce or death, loss of a job, or any one of a number of events that they consider significant. In their application interview they are asked to address these issues. Students are further requested to address any significant events that have occurred during their time of ministry training. They are encouraged to document and evaluate these occurrences during the mid-term and final evaluation parts of the program.[4] For some students this aspect of the program gives particular insight and provides them with the opportunity to confront and reintegrate past events that had been avoided. (Of course, for others, no such insights were forthcoming.) This part of the program gave new life to many people and a new understanding of the importance of memory—or the lack of it—to one's identity.

Verbatim writing

The second method of engaging memory is within verbatim writing, in which students are expected to document the effectiveness of their ministry to patients. Verbatim writing requires students to record word for word the content of pastoral conversations they have had with a patient. It is not only an art, but also a skill. Students who have not previously used this method often find it difficult to remember a conversation word for word. Most become more adept as they gain more experience. I encourage the students to make the notation 'I have forgotten' if they cannot remember any part of the conversation. What students forget is interesting and sometimes significant. These forgotten slices of conversation often prove a significant learning point. For some students the material they have 'forgotten' confronts them with painful memories which have not been dealt with and which potentially inhibit them as carers. It is not appropriate for some students to deal with these 'forgotten' memory events, but for others it proves to be a significant point in their lives and spirituality. The role of supervision is to make connections between these memory events and their influences upon students' lives, ministry, and understanding of God.[5]

THE TENSION BETWEEN CLOSENESS AND DISTANCE

This tension is illustrated in the ethic of care as it affects patient, carer, and supervisor. Care is both a challenge to security and a means for growth. Mayeroff, for example, defines caring as 'helping the other to grow' (1971, p. 5). He writes, 'I experience what I care for … as an extension of myself and at the same time as something separate from me that I respect in its own right' (1971, p. 5). For Mayeroff the common venture in caring is that of nonpossessive closeness, which recognises that the other person has inherent value and is independent of me. Noddings (1984) makes the same point about the other as an extension of the self, but gives an added dimension in conveying the powerful emotional content of this version of the ethics of care. She writes: 'The one-caring comes across to the cared-for in an attitude. Whatever she does she conveys to the cared-for that she cares … If she tends the sick, her hands are gentle with the anticipation of pain and discomfort. If she comforts the night-terrored child, her embrace shields from both terror and ridicule. She feels the excitement, pain, terror, or embarrassment of the other and commits herself to act accordingly' (Noddings 1984, p. 59). This is a moving description, but it does raise the possibility of engulfment by the other, a danger that Mayeroff is careful to avoid with his warning about parasitic relationships. Elsewhere, however, Noddings seems to recover the tension of closeness and distance, and her description of caring as a kind of releasing mothering is memorable: 'She [the caring mother] will send him [her child] into the world sceptical, vulnerable, courageous, disobedient and tenderly receptive' (Noddings 1984, p. 93).

The ethic of care highlights the tension between closeness and distance and, in a pertinent way, the issues of security and growth. Caring for people requires that we provide both security and the challenge to growth, a balance that becomes more complicated when people are facing death. There are many subtleties and complexities in delineating between offering people security and engaging in a journey of growth. Carl Nighswonger (1971) sees this journey as experienced through a series of tension-filled dramas, which lead to the fulfilment of one's journey in either peace or forlornness.[6] This is a dynamic journey, which illustrates the interconnectedness of physical, social, and emotional issues with the spiritual issues that confront people facing illness and death. The journey is complicated by what people bring to the various dramas, but in the end completion is found either in peace and fulfilment or withdrawal and depression. That is, the journey can be either one of growth and the completion of a life journey, or it can finish in hopelessness.

As a patient and a teacher I have decided to engage with my cancer while maintaining a balance between closeness and distance. As a chaplain I was deeply involved with people with cancer. My ministry allowed me to enter the lives of thousands, and at times my involvement—sometimes my over-involvement—was so deep that I imagined that I had cancer myself. But I did not, and over a period of time I learned to care deeply for people and at the same time keep the cancer at a distance. Today I have cancer. What does it mean to take ownership of my cancer as well as keeping it at a distance? I know that I need a balance of security and the challenge to grow. Normally, the cancer has equal status with the other influences in my life. It is one more conversation partner in my theological reflection. It does not dominate, but it is an influence, as are the other partners. It is not surprising that this cancer has implications for my role as an educator.

During a teaching session last year, for example, I discovered that I had been distancing my cancer and that this was just as troubling as allowing it to get too close to me. I came to realise that I had been disembodying my cancer, which was contrary to what I believed about the incarnation and integration. The experience leading to this realisation was a turning point for me in my approach to my cancer. I have come to realise that to fail to acknowledge who I am in my caring, teaching, supervising, and preaching is to do an injustice to the meaning of the incarnation. While I knew this previously, it becomes more poignant as I am faced with my terminal illness.

Can you imagine the conversation I have with my cancer? The cancer cells say, 'We're here to offer pastoral care to you.' Which means, I think, 'We have come to let you know you are finite.' Sometimes their statement is of a theological nature: 'We are here to prove that God created evil.' My response, after a long discussion, is 'I don't believe my God creates cancer.' At other times they say, 'If you do this for me, we will not multiply as quickly as we are supposed to.' My response has been, 'I am not ready to bargain with you.' But while my cancer cells are an important conversation partner there are other partners who provide a different message: my faith, the love for and from my wife Marlene, my children, family, friends, and my theological community all provoke different kinds of conversation. My choice to theologically and spiritually engage my cancer has provided new life and hope for me on this penultimate inner journey.

ISSUES FOR SUPERVISION

The tension between closeness and distance is also an issue in training for supervision. Supervision aims to effect change and growth in trainees. While the supervisor offers unfeigned warmth, acceptance, kindness, and security to the supervised, the supervisor must do more than this if the aim of supervision is to be achieved. There is often a close bond between the supervisor and the supervised. However, if the relationship is no more than this one has to question the supervisor's motives. Sometimes the supervised is so enmeshed with the life and character of the supervisor that it is difficult to differentiate between them. When this happens it is apparent that closeness and security have been the predominant influences in the relationship. Rabbi David Oler (1999) says all transferences set up false idolatrous gods and impede the growth and development of autonomy and differentiation of the supervised. He discourages 'collusion of the gods' and 'conflict of the gods' but encourages 'constructive confrontation of the gods' in order that the supervised might develop his or her own autonomy. The issue of differentiation and autonomy is vital to the growth of people intellectually, emotionally, and spiritually, and is particularly important to many who are facing death. It is my contention that in modelling the creative tension between closeness and distance in the supervisory relationship the supervised will, in turn, become better equipped not only to care for himself or herself but also become a more effective carer to those who are facing death.

The tension between caring about and receiving care

Many of those who are good at caring about others have difficulty in receiving care themselves, and this certainly was my realisation at the onset of my cancer. Once again Noddings has something interesting to say concerning caring about and receiving care. She argues that a detached 'masculine' understanding of care, which emphasises competence and responsibility, excludes the connected 'feminine' concerns for attentiveness and responsiveness. Her analysis of care, which centres on mutuality and receptivity, asserts that joy is also a basic human affect, despite the fact that conflict and guilt are inevitable in our caring. She asserts that 'caring about' versus 'caring for' sets up an ontology of joy as against an ontology of anxiety. While Noddings may be stereotyping differences between 'masculine' and 'feminine' care, the distinctions and implications are important for the tensions of giving and receiving care (Noddings 1984, pp. 16–21).

This distinction was certainly important for the friends of Henri Nouwen,[7] who were most critical of his decision to commit his life to caring for disabled people in Toronto's L'Arche Daybreak Community. Nouwen's friends were not in sympathy with his decision to leave a high-profile academic position at Yale Divinity School for one that they considered menial and beneath his gifts and abilities. Perhaps their understanding of care emphasised competence and responsibility, but not the joy and mutuality that Nouwen received from his care of people in the community. Nouwen was so moved by the depth of his spiritual experience there that he wrote a book, *Adam*, based on the life of Adam, for whom he cared (Nouwen 1997); Nouwen died in 1996 before being able to complete it.

Adam was a severely handicapped young man. He could not speak, or even move, without assistance. In the eyes of the world he was a complete nobody. And yet for Nouwen, Adam became a friend, teacher, and guide. It was Adam who led Nouwen to new insights into faith and what it means to be beloved by God. Nouwen discovered his disability through Adam and, in so doing, learnt how to receive care graciously and naturally. For Nouwen caring for Adam was a joy.

Michael Ford (1999) depicts Nouwen as both a warm and generous person and as someone who fought hard with the inner demons of insecurity and anxiety, restlessly searching for love and liberty, a wounded prophet. During his final years, Nouwen discovered a joyful freedom with a travelling circus group with whom he could forget people's expectations of him. The experience engaged his childlike wonder and his theological and spiritual wisdom in creative new ways. He came to think of the trapeze as a simple yet powerful metaphor for the spiritual life: it is about allowing oneself to let go and trusting that one will be caught. At one level Nouwen was obviously the flyer who needed to be caught and held—but at another level he was very much the catcher, in the way in which he received people unconditionally and nonjudgmentally; being present to them with a spirit that gave security and confidence, yet pointed them to something beyond.

When I reflect on this image of the flyer and the catcher, I find that most of my life has involved flying (taking risks) and catching people (pastoral care). I find it very difficult to allow myself to be caught. I have lived a satisfying life and I know I have difficulty in letting go of things and relationships that have touched me deeply. I value intimacy and the meaning that comes from that intimacy. My relationship with my wife reflects a mutuality of intimacy, integrity, and respect, which we value deeply. Our relationship has all the values that I understand to be spirituality. I know too that this is not only an issue for many who are dying, but also for their carers. And so I am not ready to be caught, even though I know its significance. A great deal of my ministry to dying people was catching them, taking men and women in my arms and cradling them. I know this act consoled and uplifted those people who were dying. I am beginning to allow myself to be caught and cared for, but I want to be a flyer and a catcher as long as I am permitted. I suspect, as time goes by, that I will be more in the position of being caught. However, if this image of the catcher is a foretaste of hope and new life, then it is something to look forward to. Nouwen said: 'Dying is trusting in the catcher. To care for the dying is to say, "Don't be afraid. Remember that you are a beloved child of God. He will be there when you make your long jump. Don't try and grab him; he will grab you. Just stretch out your arms and hands and trust, trust, trust" ' (Ford 1999, p. 224). This is a moving image of what it means to trust in someone, in this case, God. The issue of trust for the dying person is of the utmost importance. The absence of trust can lead to feelings of desolation, while its presence can provide hope and security, which is vital for the person facing death. Lack of trust is often focused in the fear that the person will be deserted physically, emotionally, and spiritually during their time of dying. Someone has said, 'Hell is where no people are,' It is crucial for many people to know and trust that they will not be deserted during this time. To know this trust of presence can allow the dying person to let go and place their trust in the presence of their God. The carer can model this trust and encourage loved ones to provide this presence during this time. I have witnessed the pain of many who have been deserted emotionally and spiritually. It is important, therefore, that this trust of presence be present in our daily living relationships in order to prepare for its continuity as we face our dying. Trust is the basis of any relationship, but it becomes of the greatest importance when we come to the end of our lives.

PASTORAL SUPERVISION

Caring for the dying is a privilege, and it is also a responsibility. To care with commitment requires a great deal of emotional and spiritual energy. Pastoral supervision addresses the delicate balance involved in being a 'wounded healer' for others (Asquith 1991). Being fully present for others, sharing in their struggles, and making use of the self in pastoral relationships results in what William Oglesby calls 'the erosion of the self' (1980, p. 196). Perhaps more than any other relationship, the pastoral relationship can set up transferences and countertransferences that require attention for the sake of both the dying person and the carer. Further, carers often develop intimate relationships that can, for many reasons, lead to emotional overinvestment and overinvolvement. I do not criticise intimacy, as it is required when dealing with the intimacy of death, but there are times when lines need to be drawn for the sake of the dying person. For instance, inappropriate overinvolvement can inhibit the dying person letting go in order to live their dying. Caring for the dying is not an easy ministry and nor should it be if we care deeply. The issue for most committed carers is not in their caring, but their difficulty in receiving care. I have stated that I have found it difficult being the patient, but I have always been receptive to supervision. Pastoral supervision not only provided me with the security I needed, but also offered feedback on my strengths and weaknesses that assisted me in placing things in perspective. I learnt through the modelling of my supervisor that I could develop deep relationships with dying people without getting overinvolved. I discovered that I could do this only as I developed intimate primary relationships outside the institution where I worked. Pastoral supervision helped me set appropriate boundaries in the pastoral relationship while at the same time recognising that, as Oglesby says, it was the relationship itself that became the source of healing for me (Oglesby 1980, p. 41).

The pastoral supervisory relationship provides the supervised with a model of self-giving love, which can set limits but also enables the supervised to experience a vital, healing relationship. I could not have cared for dying people for thirteen years without the ministry of supervision.

I have been on a wonderful journey and perhaps the most significant part of that journey has been the spiritual formation I received in caring for people with cancer. It has been the backbone of my pastoral care and supervision. Now I too have cancer, and the journey and the spiritual formation continues. It continues to be a wonderful—although sometimes sad—journey. There have been many tensions on the journey, tensions that have caused me anxiety and pain, but I must say that it has also been through these tensions that my life and faith have been enriched.

CONCLUSION

I have outlined three tensions that the spiritual care-giver will experience when caring for people who are dying. It is at the equilibrium points of these tensions that supervision focuses in order that the spiritual care-giver might not only set boundaries but also grow in understanding of the self and the other. There can be dangers in practising spiritual care without appropriate supervision. There is often a degree of subtlety required to detect the dangers inherent in these tensions, and without adequate supervision spiritual care-givers may be in danger not only of harming the dying person but also themselves.

There is value in having ongoing supervision for professional development whether you are a care-giver of the dying person or in some other setting. However, the issues for the spiritual care-giver are often intensified when caring for the dying person. Many religious denominations are beginning to see the value of supervision for the professional development of their ministers, and pressure is growing for supervisors to be trained and accredited to undertake this important task. Similar standards of training and accreditation should also apply to the supervision of spiritual care-givers in palliative care.

While I have been speaking of one-to-one supervision there is also value in developing peer supervision, where care-givers supervise and support each other in a group setting. The role of the supervisor in the group setting would be one of facilitator. I have indicated in this chapter the importance for my supervision of the use of the verbatim and case study methods in order to focus on issues for supervision. Here, the focus is on the spiritual care-giver and the issues that allowed or prevented the care-giver from providing adequate care to the dying person. I am aware that many care-givers struggle to retrieve the information required for a verbatim or case study, but it is my experience that this struggle provides a basis not only for more adequate care to the dying person but also for the ongoing professional development of the care-giver.

The ultimate outcome of ongoing supervision is that the spiritual care-giver will develop skills and insights that will eventually allow him or her to engage spontaneously and immediately in self-supervision. This does not mean the cessation of ongoing supervision for the spiritual care-giver but it does mean that the care-giver often operates at a new level of skill and insight which can only mean more adequate care for the person for whom we have been given the privilege of caring.

REFERENCES

Asquith, G. A. 1991, 'Pastoral theology and supervision: An integrative approach', *Journal of Supervision and Training in Ministry*, vol. 13, pp. 165–79.

Ford, M. 1999, *Wounded Prophet: A Portrait of Henri J. M. Nouwen*, Darton, Longman & Todd, London.

Freud, S. 1956, 'Mourning and melancholia' (1917), in S. Freud, *Collected Papers*, Hogarth Press, London, vol 4, pp. 152–70.

George, E. 1999, *In Pursuit of the Proper Sinner*, Hodder & Stoughton, London.

Le Carré, J. 1999, *The Secret Pilgrim*, Hodder & Stoughton, London.

Mayeroff, M. 1971, *On Caring*, Harper & Row, New York.

Nighswonger, C. 1971, 'Ministry to the dying as a learning encounter', *Journal of Thanatology*, vol. 1, pp. 101–8.

Noddings, N. 1984, *Caring: A Feminine Approach to Ethics and Moral Education*, University of California Press, Berkeley.

Nouwen, H. 1997, *Adam: God's Beloved*, Orbis Books, New York.

Oglesby, W. 1980, *Biblical Themes for Pastoral Care*, Abingdon, Nashville.

Oler, D. 1999, 'Pastoral supervision and operational theology', *American Journal of Pastoral Counselling*, vol.2, no. 1, pp. 3–13.

Paver, J. 1994, 'The influence of memory on ministry and spirituality', *Ministry, Society and Theology*, vol. 8, no. 2, pp. 52–67.

Thayer, N. 1985, *Spirituality and Pastoral Care*, Fortress Press, Philadelphia.

NOTES

1 For ten years I had dual responsibilities at Peter MacCallum Cancer Institute where I was Inter-Church chaplain and Director of the Clinical Pastoral Education program. For three years I was chaplain to the Palliative Care Unit at the Heidelberg Repatriation Hospital, Victoria and also a Director of a Clinical Pastoral Education program.

2 While George's work is fiction, I experienced from reading it an understanding of the meaning of self-deception, as I also experienced in John Le Carré's novel, *The Secret Pilgrim*.

3 In this collection Freud suggests that if the memory of suffering is suppressed it continues to dominate a person in unhealthy ways. Today, this is not news. However, his words suggest a dialectic of forgetting and remembering; only by remembering can we be free to act without being dominated by unconscious memory. This chapter is not advocating that carers should delve into the unconscious of the people for whom they care, but it does suggest that carers should be aware that people with cancer who are facing death can elicit in them forces which, if not dealt with, can have a deleterious effect on them as people and as carers.

4 I am aware that I could be accused of trying to change people's history at this sensitive time. I am also aware that this action could cause psychological and spiritual pain. I am not trying to change people's history, but I am encouraging them to remember their history in order that they live life more fully.

5 These methods were developed during my tenure as Director of Clinical Pastoral Education, Peter MacCallum Cancer Institute, from 1976–85. The notion of autobiography is my development, but the verbatim method has been tested over many years.

6 This journey comprises six dramas: denial or panic, catharsis or depression, bargaining or selling out, realistic hope or despair, acceptance or resignation, and fulfilment or forlornness.

7 Henri Nouwen was a priest and, as the author of twenty books, one of the most prominent Christian spiritual writers of the 1980s and 1990s.

Part 3

Developing Responses

Introduction

Previous sections have focused upon the contexts and ways in which spirituality emerges and is acted upon, and some of the experiences that result from attending to spiritual issues and possibilities. This section endeavours to draw together some of the insights from the preceding chapters and explore implications for spiritual care in palliative care settings.

First, Allan Kellehear (chapter 11) focuses key features of social and pastoral approaches to spirituality in a discussion of who should offer spiritual care. Next, Pamela McGrath (chapter 12) reviews the wealth of literature that has already been produced around the linked themes of spirituality and spiritual care, identifying key issues that emerge and illustrating how research in spirituality can provide a way forward. Her discussion of the problem of definition here is particularly helpful. The detailed referencing of this chapter is a resource for those who wish to explore the healthcare spiritual care literature further.

Chapter 13 (Bruce Rumbold) develops one of the images that has been used frequently in the preceding sections, that of dying as a quest. It explores whether there are ways in which this image will allow us to learn from the dynamics of traditional spiritualities, while resisting or revising their institutional forms. The image seems to be one that can both capture and transcend boundaries between belief systems and, while drawing upon traditional resources, keep us open to new possibilities, both individually and corporately.

Common to the three chapters is an insistence on the need for reflective practice, a note on which we exited chapter 10. Supervision, research, and social accountability, are all needed to ensure that spirituality becomes better understood yet at the same time resists capture by any particular (professional) interests. Today's talk about spirituality matters, for it keeps care human.

11

Spiritual Care in Palliative Care: Whose Job is It?

Allan Kellehear

There is a deep but hidden paradox in our understanding of spiritual care in palliative care. It is best revealed when we pursue an answer to the question of whose responsibility it is to provide this care to dying people and their families. It seems that everyone in the palliative care literature has a ready answer to this question.

Many people believe that it is chaplains and clergy in general who should take the lead in spiritual care (Charlton 1992; Speck 1993). Others believe that it should be facilitated by nursing referrals to these chaplains (Dein & Stygall 1997; Warner-Robbins & Christiana 1989). Still others believe that it is nurses who are the frontline people in palliative care and should therefore be the professional most relevant to cater for these needs (Heliker 1992; Millison & Dudley 1990). Doctors (Hamilton 1998) and social workers (Kilpatrick & Holland 1990) have also argued that they, rather than others in palliative care, are better suited to this style or type of care. There appears no shortage of volunteers for spiritual care.

But if I ask myself or my friends, or even my local car mechanic, whose responsibility is it to find meaning in my losses, my dogs, my marriage, or my work, to find God in whatever form I can, or to understand my disappointments and limitations, most of these people would say that it is my responsibility. In other words, the everyday tasks of finding meaning, of transcending suffering, and of finding something greater than myself to assist me in those tasks is my own personal challenge. The task of spiritual care is not one for my mechanic, not one for my friends, not one for my employer. All of these people may help me in this journey—sometimes consciously and deliberately, sometimes unconsciously and unintentionally—but the essential responsibility, the first step and the last step, must be mine. This is the challenge of life itself and we are born into communities so that this task may be less of a lonely one.

Yet in the palliative care literature on spirituality this recognition of the centrality of self in healthcare in general, and spiritual care in particular, seems remote, even foreign (for an exception to this trend, see Cole 1997). We consistently see spiritual care as something that we dispense, something that *we do to others* rather than something *we do with others* because this is part of what we all do. How did this situation arise?

PALLIATIVE CARE AS ACUTE CARE

Spiritual care is frequently written about as a psychological series of 'assessments' and 'interventions'. It is a verbal activity, perhaps an exercise in self-expression or a form of 'counselling' (Bradshaw 1996, p. 414). In other writing, it is listening skills that are emphasised, as if one can meaningfully speak about actions separate from contexts or personalities. The palliative care literature is clearly problem-focused, as if the usual meeting place of one's personal meaning and its usual social sources in family and community networks are always in some way alienated or dysfunctional.

Authors speak of crises at times of illness (Hay 1989) or the 'symptoms' of spiritual 'pain' (Heyse-Moore 1996), as if we were talking about some medical problem that can or, indeed, should, be addressed by an arsenal of interventions. Without a doubt the language and storylines about care are heavily borrowed from the language and culture of acute care. This approach seems so natural because such symbolism occurs in a broader context which views such language and ideas as natural. It seems that palliative care has slowly moved from a community-based approach to end-of-life care to a clinical one. In the clinical approach the emphasis and language has been on diagnosis and management, on control of symptoms, or assessment of needs.

Research has emphasised what *we* need to know to do *our* job, the identification of *problems*, and models for the solution of those problems. The professional literature on spiritual care is replete with heroic case study narratives of problems and their successful solution because of particular pastoral interventions by some palliative care professional. How do we know so much about spiritual problems when the literature is so bereft of identification and discussions of spiritual wellbeing? Does the current emphasis on medical language

(McGrath 1999) and psychological (Walter 1997) approaches in spiritual care mean that spirituality has become yet another clinical entity in palliative care?

Clearly, palliative care has come a long way from its early religious roots as a type of care offered by religious orders to the poor wayfarer and homeless (Bradshaw 1996). It has even come a long way from Cicely Saunders's original model of a type of community-based care supported by that community, existing financially and philosophically outside the conventional medical and hospital establishment (Rumbold 1998).

Lately, with its significant absorption into the mainstream of healthcare, palliative care has received substantial financial support and political interest from governments and healthcare professionals. In particular, doctors and nurses have been at the forefront of lobbying governments for increased funding and development, of developing professional societies and journals that recognise the area as a significant practice specialty, and of developing a research agenda designed for knowledge expansion and service improvements.

Today, palliative care is, without dispute, first and foremost a healthcare specialty the principal character and language of which is clinical. The emphasis is on assessment and management of health outcomes, notwithstanding that the main outcome will usually be death.

As a clinical specialism, limiting its expertise to issues of health and illness, and these principally at the end of life, there does not appear to be much of a problem. However, problems do emerge from this particular way of viewing palliative care as soon as one adds two important omissions to this vision of palliative care: first, that palliative care should, according to Cicely Saunders (1987, p. 57), apply across the lifespan of the disease from the time of diagnosis, and second, that palliative care is multidisciplinary. The second point means that not only is palliative care a type of care that is physical and psychological, but it is also care that is spiritual and social.

Both of these points—the multidisciplinary care and care that is early and late in the course of life-limiting illness—means that palliative care cannot afford to be merely clinical in its emphasis if it is to be social, spiritual, and early care. Palliative care, in this vision, becomes community care as well as clinical care. The idea of palliative care as public health has enjoyed only recent attention (Kellehear 1999; Rumbold 2000). Whatever its ultimate merits or shortcomings, however, this community-oriented approach poses at least one useful question of palliative care: who and what are its role models in healthcare?

When we examine the way in which spiritual care is discussed—in terms of preferred language and storylines—it seems that much of the discussion has adopted a rather clinical, acute care style. It has been clinical in style because the emphasis has not been on health, normality, culture, or community but on crises, problems, or professional territory and rivalry. It has been acute care in style because the emphasis has not been on community development, social networks, or how professions themselves contribute rather than alleviate problems of modernity and spirituality. The emphasis has instead been on individual interventions, professional techniques, and skills acquisition. Spirituality becomes the newest topic of inservice training, the latest argument for the professionalisation of pastoral care or nursing, or yet another criticism thrown at the medical profession.

If there were a public health approach to spiritual care, a perspective that emphasised community and took an inclusive rather than territorial approach, what would it look like?

SPIRITUALITY AND HEALTH PROMOTING PALLIATIVE CARE

I have discussed elsewhere (Kellehear 2000) the importance of viewing spirituality in terms of dimensions of need. No pithy definition of spirituality is adequate to capturing the diversity and complexity of spiritual desire. Spirituality can be understood as a desire for transcendence, a search for meaning that will take the person beyond the immediacy of his or her personal suffering. Meanings in this context help people make sense of suffering and are crucial in the development and maintenance of hope, courage, and, to some extent, personal acceptance.

I identified three sources of transcendence: situational, moral and biographical, and religious. In situational transcendence, individuals examine their bodily or immediate environmental situation and look to find sources of hope, purpose, meaning and affirmation, mutuality, connectedness, and company. These are the personal tools, as it were, to make sense of and surmount the confusion, disorientation, and anxiety of painful, difficult, and foreign physical and social experiences.

From these reflections about the immediacy of their situation other spiritual needs may emerge. Here, moral and biographical needs such as the desire for reconciliation, reunion, forgiveness, closure, or moral and social analysis may arise as a result of the confrontation with mortality. Some of these needs may resemble religious needs but they differ in important ways. Moral and biographical needs are not resolved by religious responses to them. Personal expressions of these needs—for example, prayer—are not designed to alter one's ultimate fate or relationship with God but represent satisfying personal alternatives to intellectualism for the development of hope and the restoration of morale.

Many people do have frankly religious needs. The jury is still out on the secularisation of the modern world (Bradshaw 1996) and international surveys consistently show high levels of religious belief despite low church attendance (Gallop & Proctor1982). In this context, people with life-threatening illnesses may express a desire for religious reconciliation, divine forgiveness and support, religious rites or sacraments, visits by clerics, and religious reading and discussion opportunities.

From these final lists of needs we may surmise that someone—a chaplain or cleric from the local community—might be relevant to help address these needs. In some cases, staff members of palliative care or within hospice may be valuable, especially if that person shares similar beliefs to the dying person but does not belong to the local community. Local communities can be supportive but they can also be claustrophobic and gossipy.

Many of the moral and biographical needs can entail parallel needs to visit others or to be visited by them. Sometimes—for example, in a desire to know about the possibilities of reunion in death—some form of death education and discussion with someone who is familiar with research in this area might be important. At other times and in other examples, facilitating a sense of closure may mean executing an elaborate process of gift giving and/or visitations. In all these cases, moral and biographical needs have a high proportion of social and physical action with the community and networks of the dying person.

Finally, making sense of a terminal illness, a poor prognosis, or being institutionalised in a hospice or hospital may require some discussion and reflection. This is best done with old friends or close relatives, perhaps even a lifetime partner if that person is still available and desired. Sometimes these are important opportunities for pastoral carers or social workers to spend time with these people. But at other times, even the cleaners in these institutions have been known to play valuable roles in this capacity of meaning-making.

You will note that in all these above discussions of spiritual need a connection with community and the role of action rather than simple discussion with health professionals are paramount. This community action orientation is not absolute and total. There is an important role for listening, discussion, counselling, and joint reflection with professionals. But the major role—and the major impetus to act—lies with the person with the life-threatening illness, with the self and his or her usual social world. In difficult times there is frequently much to do—friends to see, relatives to speak to, work colleagues to deal with. There are preparations to make, farewells to bid, conversations to be had, special people to call for, places to visit, gifts to make, things to think, values to clarify, embraces to find their target (Kellehear 1990).

In other words, spiritual needs have a large community-based component, which friends and relatives know is their responsibility as much as it is that of their dying member. The social self is the main actor, the person-in-the-world, who needs to act and knows they need to act. And they need to act within their own community. What are the theoretical tools for understanding this role and its facilitation?

Health promoting palliative care is a public health approach to care based upon the World Health Organization's *Ottawa Charter of Health Promotion* (Kellehear 1999). Its fundamental role is to sensitise health workers to the practical role that community development, political action, and education can bring to the provision of a healthy quality of life. The charter stresses the importance of building public policies that support health, actions that create supportive environments and strengthen community action, develop personal skills, and reorient health services.

Health promotion is, therefore, participatory. It recognises the social character of health and illness. The emphasis is frequently on education, information and policy development, and encourages all health professionals to act for the well *and* the ill. Importantly, health promotion emphasises the fact that health is everyone's responsibility, not just that of particular individuals, such as health professionals.

For a health promoting palliative care approach all this means the need to go beyond face-to-face clinical encounters. This involves the need to act while people are well, in addition to while they are close to death. It also involves the need to develop an understanding of and set of skills that are sensitive to community as well as individual needs. In these ways, employing these kinds of public health alerts we can see how a health promoting approach might address spiritual needs of the kind that I have identified in situational, moral and biographical, and religious contexts.

THE LANGUAGE OF SPIRITUAL CARE

The principal philosophical difference between frankly clinical approaches to healthcare and public health approaches is the fact that clinical approaches target disease and seek treatment to address this problem. The aim in clinical interventions is restoration of health. A public health approach, on the other hand, targets health and quality of life and seeks prevention of disease by facilitating health maintenance and harm-minimisation approaches to illness and injury.

These two approaches are not antithetical but complementary. The emphasis in public health approaches is clearly on quality-of-life issues; the clinical strategies are at the ready for when things go wrong. Health and illness are two theoretical ideas that should be understood together so that we can maximise the first to minimise the second. The concern I have is that clinical ideas seem to overpopulate the spiritual care literature. Such language and ideas do not address spiritual needs in a balanced way—in terms of health and disease, in terms of individual interventions and community work, in terms of engagement of professional help and its wise and judicious absence.

The narratives of spiritual care repeatedly employ the language of psychology, especially clinical psychology. We constantly read about counselling, about listening skills, the importance of self-expression, or the need for empathy. Sometimes we read about the therapeutic or healing value of silence, even active presence. There is a regular concern for crisis or spiritual problems. We often speak of needs and their assessment. And if assessment reveals problems beyond the spiritual we may speak in terms of referral to colleagues in other face-to-face work—in psychology or psychiatry, for example. The emphasis is typically and firmly on the person-as-individual, personal change, and professional judgment. Seldom do we hear the language of public or community health.

The language of spiritual care

Clinical	Public health
counselling	networking
listening	participation
self-expression	mutual exchange
empathy	social connection
silence	reciprocity
active presence	respectful absence
crisis/problems	health/culture
need/assessment	mutual learning
clinical referral	advocacy
person-individual	person in community
personal change	social change
professional judgment	community knowledge

It is instructive that the language of community development or of health promotion is frequently absent from discussion of spiritual care, especially given the social nature of its personal expressions and desires. There is little doubt that personal skills in working with people are of value but where are the social skills and ideas in the language of spiritual care?

If spiritual needs are community-based, forged by the community and culture from which we are shaped as individuals, where is the language of action which recognises these sources? The need to network within communities, to befriend and learn the assumptions and values of its membership and its social diversity are seldom mentioned in academic spiritual care narratives in palliative care. The idea of participation and mutual exchange with communities rather than individual 'clients' may often be simply assumed, perhaps. But this silence creates a gap in our understanding about how professional knowledge is mediated by community experiences and knowledge. The fact that knowledge of community can compete with and give context to professional knowledge is seldom given practical recognition or discussion.

How can empathy be true, rather than method acting, without some genuine social connection to the world of the individual with whom you are working? Even the absence of such experience does not always need to be met with silence or studied behavioural skills. Genuine reciprocity, in the context of personal and social differences, is an important way of making spiritual and social connections with people attempting to make sense of foreign experiences together.

There is a need for significant discussion and research about what I call 'respectful absence'. This is the reality of how spiritual concerns—situational, moral and biographical, or religious—are resolved and/or reformulated by individuals without professional help. Most of us understand the interpersonal need to protect and honour another's privacy. We acknowledge the role this plays in the support and strengthening of another person's personal safety and dignity. Respectful absence is about protecting the honour and integrity of a person's social identity and social self-image. It is also looking at ways to enhance a person's usual spiritual supports unobtrusively, without the obvious presence of a spiritual care worker. What are the normal processes, the community-based processes, of spiritual healing and sustenance and what lessons are there in those processes for professional work?

Connected to these wider issues of community is the challenge of viewing personal change and spiritual meaning in the context of the modern fragmentation of communities. How does rapid social change in modern contexts of religious diversity or cultural and political challenges to personal meaning influence or shape the modern experience of hope and despair? How does contributing to community building add to the vision and professional enhancement of spiritual care in palliative care?

SO WHOSE JOB IS IT?

I do not mean to argue that such ideas are dismissed in discussions of spiritual care. I do not even suggest that many of the questions that I raise are necessarily new ones. My observations and questions are directed at what I see as imbalances in the major storylines and languages of spiritual care in palliative care. The reasons for that imbalance may be understandable enough.

Perhaps the imbalance is due to our taken-for-granted assumptions that this work is always the basis of other more problem-oriented work that is performed in spiritual care—for individuals and communities. In this way, we tend to write and publish more about things that worry us. Some of us may feel that the bigger challenges come from particular characters or personal dilemmas.

Perhaps the imbalance of language and ideas about spiritual care comes from the fact that so much spiritual care in palliative care occurs in closed environments such as inside homes, clinics, or hospices. Perhaps the concentration of interest around counselling and listening skills has something to do with the practical value of adopting a language that most other professionals in a clinical setting can readily understand. This may make interprofessional interest and cooperation easier to establish and maintain.

Whatever reasons are truly implicated one practical consequence of a move away from social languages and practices is the impression that perhaps spiritual care values its links with other professions more than it does its links with community. If its role models are clinical some may surmise that spiritual care values its role in disease more than its role in health, values its professional resemblance to clinical psychology rather than public health.

If spiritual care is defined as care of person-in-community rather than person-in-bed I wonder how many professions would be eager to answer the question of who is responsible for that care in their own favour? The skills of health promotion—in particular of community development, community care, and the facilitation of social change—are not skills or experiences appropriate to, or readily promoted in, institutional contexts.

Furthermore, few professionals have the time for these kinds of work outside or within their usual clinical responsibilities. But by defining down spirituality, by reducing it to problems, and by addressing these problems with psychological interventions, is to sell the task of spiritual care well short of its complexities and responsibilities. It is also to define the task of spiritual care as a direct-service task. Defined in that way, when we think of the question of whose job it is to supply that care, we automatically think in terms of professional care instead of—more correctly—community care.

So if the task of any spiritual care must include a commitment to community in a participatory capacity, as well as to a commitment to problem solving by the bedside, a commitment to prevention as well as to intervention during times of distress, a commitment to understanding the primacy of the social self rather than professional expertise, the answer to whose job it is lies at the door of which professions or nonprofessionals are able to meet those commitments.

Clearly, spiritual care is directed at different dimensions of human need— situational, moral and biographical, and religious meaning. These meanings find their beginnings and their nurturance within contexts of the social spaces we have come to call community—cultures and social networks that cradle and give rise to individual, personal meanings. Successful health promotion—indeed, successful spiritual promotion—is about recognition and work within those contexts and origins.

Interpreted in this public health way, spiritual care is self-care that is everyone's responsibility. The job of spiritual care, then, can only really be understood in terms of a division of labour that crosses a number of issues, sites, and times. Spiritual care is more than conversation or being there to answer spiritual questions. It is also about participation and guardianship of a community's search for meaning in life, death, and loss. In the end, good spiritual care like good healthcare itself, is about recognition of the limits of individual professional practice.

Millison and Dudley (1990, p. 77) remarked that 'spiritual care is too critical to be left to clergy'. Yet the professional and epistemological irony is that spiritual care is too broad to be left to clinicians. A review of the current literature suggests that in the race to add spiritual care to the ambitions of certain clinical professions the first casualties of that race appear to be the definitions of spiritual care itself. These are frequently downsized and narrowed in ways convenient to their clinical advocates. Spiritual care becomes psychological gossamer to the ongoing development of palliative care as clinical work. But, as I have argued, this is neither true of the nature of spiritual care nor the interdisciplinary vision of palliative care.

The only professionals who are able to take up the challenge of spiritual care in palliative care are those who can legitimately mount and sustain a case for ongoing community involvement. They are also people whose education reflects an understanding of diverse spiritual and religious traditions. And they are people who display an understanding and practice that works the spaces between the tension that is spiritual health and distress in whichever way these are defined by the individuals themselves.

Such characteristics point to those in pastoral care or social work but they do not necessarily do so. Within these occupational groups the influence of individualising traditions is also alive and well and it does not follow that a social and health promoting perspective will be important to everyone within those occupations. In community health nursing, for example, there is a strong tradition of public health practice and it may be that this occupational group should take its place within palliative care. Perhaps they will be the occupational group most likely to take up the serious social challenge of spiritual care in all its relevant sites and dimensions.

The answer to the question 'whose job is it?' must always be linked to how one defines the job itself. During this time, when palliative care is still work-ing out its identity within a clinically oriented healthcare system, it remains unclear whose job it is to participate in a health promoting spiritual care. But if this spiritual care is not to be merely another style of psychological care in yet another custodial setting, those who would wish to inherit its mantle will need to grasp its essential cultural and community meanings. In this way, as Rumbold argues (2000), the future of spiritual care and the question of its credibility may well lie with its affinities and links to public and community health. In the meantime we can wait and see. And act.

REFERENCES

Bradshaw, A. 1996, 'The spiritual dimension of hospice: The secularisation of an ideal', *Social Science and Medicine*, vol. 43, no. 3, pp. 409–19.

Charlton, R. C. 1992, 'Spiritual needs of the dying and bereaved—views from the United Kingdom and New Zealand', *Journal of Palliative Care*, vol. 8, no. 4, pp. 38–40.

Cole, R. 1997, 'Meditation in palliative care—a practical tool for self-management', *Palliative Medicine*, vol. 11, pp. 411–13.

Dein, S. & Stygall, J. 1997, 'Does being religious help or hinder coping with chronic illness? A critical review of the literature', *Palliative Medicine*, vol. 11, pp. 291–8.

Gallop, G. & Proctor, W. 1982, *Adventures in Immortality*, Souvenir Press, London.

Hamilton, D. G. 1998, 'Believing in patients' beliefs: Physician attunement to the spiritual dimension as a positive factor in patient healing and health', *American Journal of Hospice and Palliative Care*, September/October, pp. 276–9.

Hay, M. W. 1989, 'Principles in building spiritual assessment tools', *American Journal of Hospice Care*, September/October, pp. 25–31.

Heliker, D. 1992, 'Reevaluation of nursing diagnosis: Spiritual distress', *Nursing Forum*, vol. 27, no. 4, pp. 15–20.

Heyse-Moore, L. H. 1996, 'On spiritual pain in the dying', *Mortality*, vol. 1, no. 3, pp. 297–315.

Kellehear, A. 1990, *Dying of Cancer: The Final Year of Life*, Harwood Academic, London.

—— 1999, *Health Promoting Palliative Care*, Oxford University Press, Melbourne.

—— 2000, 'Spirituality and palliative care: A model of needs', *Palliative Medicine*, vol. 14, pp. 149–55.

Kilpatrick, A. C. & Holland, T. P. 1990, 'Spiritual dimensions of practice', *Clinical Supervisor*, vol. 8, no. 2, pp. 125–39.

McGrath, P. 1999, 'Exploring spirituality through research', *Progress in Palliative Care*, vol. 7, no. 1, pp. 3–9.

Millison, M. B. & Dudley, J. R. 1990, 'The importance of spirituality in hospice work: A study of hospice professionals', *Hospice Journal*, vol. 6, no. 3, pp. 63–78.

Rumbold, B. 1989, 'Spiritual dimensions in palliative care', in P. Hodder & A. Turley (eds), *The Creative Option in Palliative Care*, Melbourne City Mission, Melbourne, pp. 110–27.

—— 1998, 'Implications of mainstreaming hospice into palliative care services', in J. Parker & S. Aranda (eds), *Palliative Care: Explorations and Challenges*, Maclennan & Petty, Sydney, pp. 3–20.

—— 2000, 'Pastoral care and public health', *Ministry, Society and Theology*, vol. 14, no. 1, pp. 57–61.

Saunders, C. 1987, 'What's in a name?', *Palliative Medicine*, vol. 1, pp. 57–61.

Speck, P. 1993, 'Spiritual issues in palliative care', in D. Doyle, G. W. C. Hanks, & N. MacDonald (eds), *Oxford Textbook of Palliative Medicine*, Oxford University Press, Oxford, pp. 517–25.

Walter, T. 1997, 'The ideology and organisation of spiritual care: Three approaches', *Palliative Medicine*, vol. 11, pp. 21–30.

Warner-Robbins, G. & Christiana, N. M. 1989, 'The spiritual needs of persons with AIDS', *Family Community Health*, vol. 12, no. 2, pp. 43–51.

12

New Horizons in Spirituality Research

Pamela McGrath

> Research is to see what everyone else has seen and to think
> what no one else has thought.

Albert Szent-Gyorgi, Hungarian Nobel laureate

The challenge of creating the space within the modern healthcare system to address spiritual issues is fundamental to the role of hospice and palliative care (O'Connor 1988). The concept of spirituality includes the individual's quest for meaning, either through religion or a simple existential questioning of the events of everyday life (Cawley 1997). The spiritual dimension is interpreted as the need for meaning, purpose, and fulfilment in life, which includes hope, the will to live, and, for some, a relationship to a transcendent power (Burkhardt & Nagai-Jacobson 1985; Harrison 1993; Soeken & Carson 1987). A spiritual discourse not only informs the holistic response to patient and family care (Emblen & Halstead 1993; Reed 1987; Saunders 1994; Sims 1987; Smith et al. 1993), but is also documented as a key factor that inspires and drives the hospice reform movement (Cassidy 1991; Du Boulay 1984; James & Field 1992; McGrath 1997a, 1998a). Consequently, preserving the spiritual dimension of organisation and care is essential to ensuring the integrity of hospice and palliative care service provision.

It was hoped that the reformist hospice movement would encourage an environment where a higher priority would be given to spirituality in a system that had long avoided the spiritual component of care (Millison 1995; O'Connor 1988). However, in the twenty-first century, with the mainstreaming of palliative care, the challenge of protecting the spiritual vision and ideology is increasingly threatened by the encroachment of bureaucratisation and routinisation (James & Field 1992; McGrath, 1997a). One strategy, it will be argued, for meeting the challenge of protecting the compassionate, holistic, and democratic hospice vision is to use the medium of research. Legitimisation of the spiritual discourse through research is essential if it is to command the 'knowledge/power' (Foucault 1972, 1973, 1980) to be integrated appropriately into the mainstream biomedical discourse.

Historically, the knowledge base in relation to spiritual issues has predominantly been recorded in the anecdotal and inspired philosophical writings of the charismatic leaders in hospice care. It has only been in recent years that aspects of the spiritual discourse have been explored through the medium of academic research (Fry 2000). Unfortunately, because of the prevailing positivist, scientific discourse of modern Western healthcare, the reliance on anecdotal literature has contributed to the situation where notions of spirituality continue to be marginalised as unsubstantiated claims of 'soft talk' (McGrath 1999). The esoteric discourse of spirituality is not legitimated in a biomedical healthcare system driven by epistemological reverence of quantitative, supposedly objective, data and evidence-based assessment of outcomes. As Oldnall (1996) argues, spirituality has been neglected in recent times as models of healthcare have relied on a biopsychosocial model of humanity. In part the problem is related to the difficulty of defining spirituality and analysing what remains an essentially intangible subject (Cawley 1997; White 2000). The way forward is to document aspects of the spiritual discourse through sophisticated qualitative methodologies so that research findings are available to inform the wider healthcare community, to affirm the importance of the spiritual discourse, and to ensure that those in hospice and palliative care disciplines benefit from the disciplined reflection generated by insights from research.

Thus, the central argument for this chapter is that establishing creative research programs on spirituality—albeit a challenging task—is the *sine qua non* of protection for hospice ideology and vision. Examples will be provided of viable research programs that are going some way to meeting this need. Firstly, however, it is important to explore the obstacles to the development of such research programs in order to set the context for understanding the challenges involved in researching this previously ignored dimension.

THE IGNORED DIMENSION

Dubbed by Soeken and Carson (1986) the 'ignored dimension', the loud silence on spirituality research has been an ongoing theme in the literature (Chapman 1986; Forbes 1994; Kaye & Robinson 1994; McGrath 1997a;

Ross 1994; Stepnick & Perry 1992; Stiles 1990). The reasons for the lack of attention to research into spirituality are complex, involving such issues as barriers to funding, epistemological concerns, and definitional problems (for full discussion of these issues, see McGrath 1999).

Barriers to funding

Research is a skilled, labour-intensive, time-consuming activity that requires adequate funding for success. Historically, funding for health research in Australia has principally been for positivist, empirical projects that reflect the biomedical conceptual framework (Colquhoun & Kellehear 1996). In short, the scientific method is presently the arbiter of what is real and what can be known in healthcare (McNeill 1998). A cursory glance at any list of successful grant applications from mainstream funding organisations provides conclusive evidence that the research dollar goes, for the most part, to reductionist, hypothetico-deductively driven, biomedical research. Funding for psychosocial research is the exception rather than the rule (Good 1990) and grant monies for work on spirituality are notable for their uniqueness. One such exception, funding from the Queensland Cancer Fund for research exploring the importance of the notion of spiritual pain in palliative care, will be discussed in detail later in this chapter.

In the highly competitive milieu of funding rounds for research programs, the rewards for reductionist science are self-perpetuating because well-established programs, with successful track records built on previous funding, are more likely to attract further grants (Little 1995; McNeill 1993, 1998). Fledgling or tentative programs, especially those with innovative methodologies, will find it difficult to obtain funding (Little 1995). Unfortunately, most of the grant applications in relation to research on spirituality will be in this position.

As there is a direct relationship between academic research and the knowledge base for Western healthcare, the result of such funding policies is the marginalisation or silencing of a discourse on spirituality within the healthcare academic literature. Referred to by Fox (1995) as the 'politics of health talk', the sociological processes associated with the power of funding bodies have much to do with the construction of reality in the health arena. In a reinforcing Kuhnian (Kuhn 1970) cycle of marginalisation, the void of research on spirituality silences this notion within mainstream professional texts, which in turn means that the notions are less likely to be absorbed into mainstream health discourse. The sequelae is that spirituality will not be given priority as an appropriate topic for research. In short, limited research on spirituality discourages consistent and respectful inclusion of such notions within the belief structure of health research and practice.

Epistemological concerns

The problems with funding are exacerbated by epistemological and methodological concerns associated with the construction of knowledge in relation to spirituality. Not only is the subject of spirituality difficult to place on the research agenda, but the sophisticated qualitative methodologies necessary for such research also are not user friendly for mainstream peer review. Traditionally, healthcare has been reluctant to accept qualitative research (Boulton & Fitzpatrick 1994; White 2000). At the core of the problem is the hegemony of the positivist, quantitative methodologies of scientific healthcare research, which are not suited to creative or useful research on spirituality (McGrath 1999).

As evidenced by the volume of papers delivered at the recent World Congress on Psycho-oncology, Melbourne, 2000, psychosocial research is on the ascendancy as a voice to balance the prior exclusive concern with physiologically driven, reductionist scientific research. Increasingly, the focus is shifting from 'body as machine' (Finkler 1991) to a more holistic approach, but this is still a far cry from including an existential or spiritual dimension. Much psychosocial research is completed under the banner of behavioural and social science which, as the name suggests, seeks scientific legitimacy through attempts to measure and quantify (Fahlberg & Fahlberg 1991). Such science is predicated on notions of measurable, empirical realism that assert that only what is observed actually exists (Armstrong 1978a; 1978b). As Koenig et al. (1999) clearly state, the gold standard for this area is still the 'rigorous standards required by the scientific community'. As a nonquantifiable dimension, research on spirituality does not fit comfortably or appropriately into such limited methodological thinking. As noted by White (2000), 'something as essentially intangible and unmeasurable as spirituality can easily be neglected or dismissed'. What is needed is a move towards naturalistic, qualitative approaches that aim 'to make sense of, or interpret, phenomena in terms of the meanings people bring to them' (Denzin & Lincoln 1994).

Definitional problems

A confounding problem, typical for early researchers and still evident in some work in the area, has been the conflation of the notion of religion with the concept of spirituality. One reason for this has been the pressure to quantify, as religiosity was a useful research measurement variable that could be clearly defined through such quantifiable indices as church attendance, religious rituals, and office bearers. However, the definitional confusion was also caused by lack of metaphysical clarity, as religion was simplistically conceived of as the only obvious expression of transcendent meaning-making (McGrath 1999). The tautological reasoning was that, as many individuals express their spirituality through their religion, spirituality must be religious. Although metaphysical or religious beliefs can inform spirituality for some individuals, there is a clear distinction between spirituality and the concept of religion (O'Connor et al. 1997).

The definition of religion emphasises an organised system of faith, beliefs, worship, and practices that nurture a relationship with a superior being, divine force or supreme power (Emblen 1992; Dombeck & Karl 1987; Murray & Zentner 1985). Religiosity is the expression of faith or belief in a higher power through rituals or practices of a particular religion or denomination (O'Connor et al. 1997). Spirituality, however, is an abstract and elusive term and, as yet, there is a lack of an agreed definition in the literature (Meraviglia 1999). Preliminary definitions indicate that spirituality is broader than religion and relates to the universal quest to make sense out of existence (Highfield 1992; Nagai-Jacobson & Burkhardt 1989), a characteristic of human 'being' (Frankl 1973; Saunders 1981). In essence it is 'the organising centre of people's lives', which may or may not be religiously informed (Hodder & Turley 1989). Spirituality is as much about a connection with the ordinary as it is about the transcendent and embraces meaning-making in relation to other people, personal being, and material nature (Benson 1997; Emblen 1992; Barnard 1988). The assumption is that every person is spiritual and deals with questions of meaning, existence, and ethics: the expression of spirituality as meaning-making is not restricted to a religious or denominational context (O'Connor et al. 1997). There are myriad forms that an individual's spirituality can take in the context of today's atheistic, materialistic, pluralistic, and multicultural society (McGrath 1999).

An important caveat to this discussion is that spirituality is not seen as restricted to individuals. Collectives display a spiritual dimension; this is amply seen in the important role of spirituality evident in hospice discourse and practice (Doyle et al. 1993; Maddocks 1990; Munley 1983; Saunders et al. 1981; Siebold 1992). Based on an understanding of the centrality of personal quests for meaning in serious illness, compassionate hospice spirituality seeks to create a respectful and nonjudgmental space for patients and their families through the provision of caring relationships that promote interpersonal bonding (Bellingham et al. 1989; Cawley 1997; Munley 1983). Essentially, hospice spiritual care-giving is about the ability to enter into the world of others and respond with feeling (Millison & Dudley 1992).

However, it is important to note that, although the dichotomy between spirituality and religion can be clearly drawn and broad statements can tentatively be made about the nature of spirituality, insufficient research is available to make exact definitions. Indeed, the research that does exist suggests that the meaning of the term 'spirituality' is presently in flux (Mahoney & Graci 1999). The definitional uncertainty becomes problematic in the competitive world of research grants, where review panels are not familiar with the inductive nature of qualitative methodologies and have expectations of definitional clarity that is associated with hypothetico-deductive research. At a time when the challenge of research is to explore the very concept of spirituality itself, definitions are counterproductive as they inscribe meaning and bring closure to the construction of concepts (McGrath, 1999). Conceptually, spirituality cannot be understood as an independent entity to be measured and recorded. Researchers need to be open to the plethora of ways that individuals construct meaning from their existence by integrating the many sociocultural discourses to which they are exposed.

Researching spirituality

The obstacles to research on spirituality are real but not insurmountable. Assuming that funding can be obtained and research completed, the question then becomes one of the purpose and value of research in this area: what type of information can be obtained from research on spirituality and how is it useful? This question will be answered by a short review of topic areas from research published through international peer review, followed by a more detailed exploration of two recent projects. Mindful that the notions of hospice and palliative care originated in a spiritually inspired, charismatic, reformist movement, the detailed discussions will provide the opportunity to affirm the need to view spiritual issues at the organisational level, rather than just as an individual dynamic. Integrated into the detailed discussion of the selected projects will be examples of recommendations for practice arising out of such research. Such recommendations will provide insights on the vital importance of using findings from research on spirituality to ensure quality practice in hospice/palliative care.

A brief overview

To date, there is a limited but developing international research literature on this topic. By way of example, the research presently available touches on the spiritual dimensions of specific diagnostic groups such as HIV/AIDS (Demi et al. 1997; Pace & Stables 1997; Saynor 1988; Sherman 1996; Woods & Ironson 1999), myocardial infarction (Walton 1999), and cancer (Abraham et al. 1996; Kaczorowski 1989). It also explores the connection with grief (Kazanjian 1997), documents aspects of spiritual care (Babler 1997; Charlton 1992; Enquist et al. 1997; Harrington 1995; Kirschling & Pittman 1989; Messenger & Roberts 1994; Mickley et al. 1998; Millison & Dudley 1992; O'Connor et al. 1997; White 2000; Reese & Brown 1997; Taylor et al. 1995, 1997), looks at educational issues (Bradshaw 1997; Narayanasamy 1993), links spirituality to better physical and mental health (Courcey 1999; Fry 2000; Fryback & Reinert 1999; Mountain & Muir 2000; Swinney et al. 2001; Weiner et al. 2001), explores religious and metaphysical diversity (McGrath 1998b; McGrath & Newell 2001), and provides continuing work on maintaining the hospice vision (McGrath, 1997b; 1998c; O'Connell, 1996; Walter, 1997). It is important to note, however, that the quality of such a list of research is variable, ranging from well thought-out projects to examples of researchers conflating religiosity and spirituality and using inappropriate methodological approaches. However, the indications are that there is a growing recognition that qualitative approaches can provide valuable insights into less observable aspects of the human experience (Boulton & Fitzpatrick 1994; White 2000).

An example of research on organisational spirituality

The first detailed example is that of research conducted on an Australian Buddhist community-based hospice, Karuna Hospice Service (KHS). The full details are available both in book form (McGrath 1998c) and truncated descriptions in journal articles (McGrath 1997a, 1997b, 1998a, 1998b). The research focus was on describing the unique factors associated with KHS that gave it such a reputation for a service of excellence. The research task was to use a postmodern *episteme* informed by notions of discourse to explore the social construction of the reality of KHS through an examination of its talk or discourse. This talk was captured through open-ended interviews with a range of participants associated with the hospice, audiorecorded, and analysed thematically.

The central finding that emerged from this study indicated that a respect for a spiritual way of thinking and acting was *the* central notion energising the work of this hospice. This is a particularly significant finding in view of the fact that the research focus was on the question of the uniqueness of this organisation and did not posit spirituality as a specific issue to be explored. Spiritual talk, however, was found to be the connecting thread that linked all the participants' discussions about the work of this hospice, whether it was concerned with clients, other organisational members, or relationships with the wider community. This finding did not include any measurement or proof of the existence of the spiritual dimension but, rather, recorded the significance to those associated with KHS of a collective respect for altruistic, transcendent meaning-making. It was this shared commitment by all organisational members to a spiritual way of seeing the world that surfaced as the factor defining KHS's difference. As it was the talk about spirituality, not spirituality itself, that was recorded in this research there was no need to prove or measure. The significant point is that, through the application of postmodern notions of discourse, the importance of spirituality can be accessed by research, made discussable, and integrated within the knowledge base of healthcare provision. At that stage in their organisational development, notions of spirituality were as real and as important to members of KHS as was scientific biomedicine in their construction of reality. It was this commitment to a spiritual way of seeing and talking that contributed greatly to their reputation for excellence.

The dangers associated with success for the original hospice grassroots reform movement are the processes of bureaucratisation and routinisation that set in, as a result of ties for funding and legitimation with mainstream health (Siebold 1992; James & Field 1992). The benefits of success such as funding and referrals from established biomedical institutions bring with them demands, pressures, and compromises that threaten to undermine the spiritual ethos that energises hospice ideology and practice. The research on this subject that does exist indicates that maintaining hospice spirituality and singleness of purpose in the face of such mainstream demands, which is difficult at best (Abel 1986; Clark 1993; James & Field 1992), is seen as one of the important tasks ahead for the hospice movement (Wald et al. 1980).

Recommendations from the research on KHS provide insights on ways to address this significant problem. First, the research indicates that, for one hospice (KHS) at least, a strong commitment to a spiritual discourse within the organisation does offer—if only to some degree—resistance to the demands of routinisation. The findings indicate that it is important for hospice organisations to openly acknowledge and value their spiritual discourse as protective and significant. The suggestion is not that this is an easy process but, rather, it is a struggle to 'maintain the angst'. Second, the findings indicate that incorporating spirituality as a criterion in staff selection is important in ensuring a continuing respect for a spiritual ethos within the organisation. Last, it was found that, by giving priority to the struggle to maintain a spiritual way of thinking and talking, the organisation will act as a 'discursive magnet' attracting like-minded individuals (workers and clients) who will, in turn, support the spiritual ethos. The recommendations can be summed up in the words of one participant who stated, 'So I think what Karuna has done is to put it on the agenda, to give spirituality some acknowledgment and say this is an important factor.'

This example has been included in the discussion to emphasise that, as research progresses in the area of spirituality, it is vitally important to embrace an organisational, as well as personal, perspective.

AN EXAMPLE OF RESEARCH ON PERSONAL SPIRITUALITY

The second study for detailed discussion focuses on the notion of meaning-making, with its mirror-opposite, spiritual pain, for the individual, be they patient, carer, or survivor. This qualitative study, the first of its kind funded by the Queensland Cancer Fund, is informed by a phenomenological methodology. Indepth, nondirective interviews are conducted with a range of individuals coping with the implications of serious illness, including hospice patients, the significant others who care for them, and survivors of cancer. The interviews are audiorecorded, transcribed verbatim, and thematically analysed using the free node system provided by the NUD*IST computer package. The intent of the study is to explore ways in which individuals who are facing serious illness construct meaning from their experience and, through that process, to examine the relevance of the notion of spiritual pain for palliative care. A subsection of the study explores hospice health professionals' understanding of their patients' issues in relation to meaning-making or spirituality.

Although the project is still in progress, preliminary data reveal insights with implications for palliative care practice and for future directions in research. Two issues have been chosen for the purpose of this discussion: interconnectedness as a vital ingredient in spirituality and the need for a new language on spirituality.

When asked to talk about the meaning they were making out of their experience with serious illness, all of the participants spoke in detail about their connections with their family and friends, their home, their work, and their leisure. Predominantly, the sense they were making out of their experience was couched in terms of how they were connected to life in the here and now, rather than in philosophical or theological frameworks. Although there were exceptions (McGrath & Newell 2001), the majority of participants expressed their spirituality singularly in terms of what they valued highly in their every-day or normal existence, not in terms of adherence to metaphysical beliefs. As one participant summed up the situation, 'No great belief in religion but a belief in life.' The richness of experience and meaning individuals reported from their everyday existence was contrasted to the spiritual pain of loneliness and disconnection experienced in the institutional hospital setting of curative medicine. Reflecting on the possibility of suicidal ideation, one participant noted: 'In hospital you are disconnected from everything and my family were not there ... I wasn't saying, oh, I could die right now. But I was sort of saying to myself, I can understand how with separation your sense of *it is all right!* just goes!' In short, *the* most important aspect of spirituality emerging from the data is the intimate connection with home and friends.

For many of the participants there was a sense in which it was difficult for them to express with clarity their ideas about their individual spirituality, espe-cially when talking about notions of transcendence. As one participant summed up the situation, 'There probably is the words but, I don't know, sometimes I ... ahhhh ... struggle a bit with saying how I feel.' Despite the shared struggle with expressing ideas, there was a remarkable similarity in the notions participants were trying to conceptualise. Thus, the initial language texts from the study strongly indicate the need for the development of a new language of spirituality. The language needs to be developed through a process of active listening to the notions that individuals are trying to express. Qualitative research is an excellent tool for such a process. As a demonstration of this process, two examples are pro-vided here of concepts that have arisen through the study. The first, 'uncertainty comfort', resembles the notion of faith for those with strong religious beliefs but is expressed by individuals who view life from an atheistic or agnostic lens. The core idea is that individuals can accept the uncertainty of not being able to know the answers to ultimate questions or metaphysical conundrums about the universe without that uncertainty having a negative impact on their meaning-making or quality of life. The inability to know is accepted with a faithlike humility. As one participant stated, 'I haven't got any answers [laughs]. I guess I've just accepted life for what it is.'

The second concept is that of 'atheistic spirituality'. It has become increas-ingly obvious from the data that the religious/atheistic dichotomy is far too simplistic and arbitrary to be conceptually useful for the subtlety of spirituality talk. For many, although the statements about not being religious were emphatic, the statements were constructed in such a way that, at the same time as denying religion, participants were communicating a reverence for life, other people, and transcendence. Typical examples are, 'No, no, we're not religious at all. You know I think my wife and I believe in—do unto others—but that is just a way of living', or, 'I think religion is about the ten commandments, that to me is how I have been brought up, what I believe. Therefore I don't need to sort of like proclaim my love to some all powerful being.' The development of a new language, both lay and academic, would go some way to facilitating private and public dialogue on these important issues.

Recommendations from the research

The preliminary findings from this research have clear pragmatic implications. First and foremost, the indications are that the most important spiritual response for patients and their carers is to ensure that they are able to remain, where possible, in the comfort of their own homes surrounded by their intimate network of family and friends. This is an area where actions speak louder than words. Primarily, individuals do not need to talk with counsellors in an institutional setting about their intimate world outside the hospital, rather, they need active, multidisciplinary support to remain in their own home as long as possible. An informed spiritual response is predominantly about the provision of choice through the development of community-based hospice and healthcare services.

Second, the findings indicate that only a minority will find religiously informed language useful for expressing their spirituality. There is a growing need for a new language of spirituality that can be shared by the broad spectrum of individuals along the continuum of metaphysical and theological uncertainty. Qualitative research methodologies have a vital role to play in meeting such a challenge.

CONCLUSION

As outlined in this chapter, spirituality is *the* vital dimension of hospice and palliative care that informs and energises at both an organisational and an individual level. However, at present, the significance of this dimension is not reflected in the knowledge base of healthcare. Marginalised as soft talk suitable only for anecdotal rumination, spirituality is yet to command respect as a topic for serious academic deliberation and research. There is a loud silence on the issue in the texts that educate the majority of our healthcare professionals. It has been argued in this paper that one important *modus operandi* for legitimating spiritual concerns and integrating talk of spirituality into the mainstream health discourse is to foster a research subculture in this area. The hope and expectation is that the findings from well-constructed projects using innovative qualitative methodologies will go some way to protecting the compassionate hospice vision and will place spirituality firmly on the healthcare agenda.

REFERENCES

Abel, E. 1986, 'The hospice movement: Institutionalising innovation', *International Journal of Health Services*, vol. 16, no. 1, pp. 71–85.

Abraham, J. et al. 1996, 'The impact of a hospice consultation team on the care of veterans with advanced cancer', *Journal of Pain and Symptom Management*, vol. 12, no. 1, pp. 23–31.

Armstrong, D.1978a, *A Theory of Universals: Universals and Scientific Realism*, vol. 11, Cambridge University Press, Cambridge.

—— 1978b, *Nominalism and Realism: Universals and Scientific Realism*, vol. 1, Cambridge University Press, Cambridge.

Babler, J. 1997, 'A comparison of spiritual care provided by hospice social workers, nurses and spiritual care professionals', *Hospice Journal*, vol. 12, no. 4, pp. 15–27.

Barnard, D. 1988, 'Love and death: Existential dimensions of physicians' difficulties with moral problems', *Journal of Medicine and Philosophy*, vol. 13, pp. 393–409.

Bellingham, R. et al. 1989, 'Connectedness: Some skills for spiritual health', *American Journal of Health Promotion*, vol. 4, no. 1, pp. 18–31.

Benson, H. 1997, *Timeless Healing*, Simon & Schuster, New York.

Bishop, R. 1999, 'Addressing issues of self-determination and legitimation in Kaupapa Maori research', in B. Webber (ed.), *He Paepae Korero: Research Perspective in Maori Education*, New Zealand Council for Educational Research, Wellington.

Boulton, M. & Fitzpatrick, R. 1994, 'Quality in qualitative research', *Critical Public Health*, vol. 5, no. 3, pp. 19–26.

Bradshaw, A. 1997, 'Teaching spiritual care to nurses: An alternative approach', *International Journal of Palliative Nursing*, vol. 3, no. 1, pp. 51–7.

Burkhardt, M. & Nagai-Jacobson, M. 1985, 'Dealing with spiritual concerns of clients in the community', *Journal of Community Health Nursing*, vol. 2, pp. 191–8.

Cassidy, S. 1991, *Sharing the Darkness: The Spirituality of Caring*, Orbis Books, New York.

Cawley, N. 1997, 'Towards defining spirituality: An exploration of the concept of spirituality', *International Journal of Palliative Care Nursing*, vol. 3, no. 1, pp. 31–6.

Chapman, L. 1986, 'Spiritual health: A component missing from health promotion', *American Journal of Health Promotion*, vol. 1, no. 1, pp. 38–41.

Charlton, R. 1992, 'Spiritual need of the dying and bereaved: Views from the United Kingdom and New Zealand', *Journal of Palliative Care*, vol. 8, no. 4, pp. 38–40.

Clark, D. (ed.) 1993, *The Future of Palliative Care: Issues of Policy and Practice*, Open University Press, Buckingham.

Colquhoun, D. & Kellehear, A. 1996, *Health Research in Practice, Personal Experiences, Public Issues*, vol. 2, Chapman & Hall, London.

Courcey, K. 1999, *Religiosity and Health: The Scientific Review of Alternative Medicine*, vol. 3, no. 2, pp. 70–4.

Demi, A. et al. 1997, 'Coping strategies used by HIV infected women', *Omega*, vol. 35, no. 4, pp. 377–91.

Denzin, N. & Lincoln, Y. (eds) 1994, *Handbook of Qualitative Research*, Sage, London.

Dombeck, M. & Karl, J. 1987, 'Spiritual issues in mental health care', *Journal of Religion and Health*, vol. 26, pp. 183–97.

Doyle, D., Hanks, G., & Macdonald, N. (eds) 1993, *Oxford Textbook of Palliative Medicine*, Oxford Medical Publications, Oxford.

Du Boulay, S. 1984, *Cicely Saunders, Founder of the Modern Hospice Movement*, Hodder & Stoughton, London.

Emblen, J. 1992, 'Religion and spirituality defined according to current use in nursing literature', *Journal of Professional Nursing*, vol. 8, no. 1, pp. 41–7.

——— & Halstead, L. 1993, 'Spiritual needs and interventions: Comparing the views of patients, nurses and chaplains', *Clinical Nurse Specialist*, vol. 7, no. 4, pp. 175–82.

Enquist, D. et al. 1997, 'Occupational therapists' beliefs and practices with regard to spirituality and therapy', *American Journal of Occupational Therapy*, vol. 51, no. 3, pp. 173–80.

Fahlberg, L. & Fahlberg, L. 1991, 'Exploring spirituality and consciousness with an expanded science: Beyond the ego with empiricism, phenomenology, and contemplation', *American Journal of Health Promotion*, vol. 5, no. 4, pp. 273–81.

Finkler, K. 1991, *Physicians at Work, Patients in Pain: Biomedical Practice and Patient Response in Mexico*, Westview Press, Oxford.

Forbes, E. 1994, 'Spirituality, aging and the community-dwelling care giver and care recipient', *Geriatric Nursing*, vol. 15, no. 6, pp. 297–302.

Foucault, M. 1972, *The Archaeology of Knowledge*, Routledge, London.

——— 1973, *The Birth of the Clinic*, Vintage, New York.

——— 1980, *Power/Knowledge*, Pantheon, New York.

Fox, N. 1995, *Postmodernism, Sociology and Health*, Open University Press, Buckingham.

Frankl, V. 1973, *The Doctor and the Soul*, Vintage, New York.

Fry, P. 2000, 'Religious involvement, spirituality and personal meaning for life: Existential predictors of psychological wellbeing in community-residing and institutional care elders', *Aging and Mental Health*, vol. 4, no. 4, pp. 375–87.

Fryback, P. & Reinert, B. 1999, 'Spirituality and people with potentially fatal diagnosis', *Nursing Forum*, vol. 34, no. 1, pp. 13–22.

Good, B. 1990, *Medicine, Rationality, and Experience: An Anthropological Perspective*, Cambridge University Press, Cambridge.

Harrington, A. 1995, 'Spiritual care: What does it mean to RNs?', *Australian Journal of Advanced Nursing*, vol. 12, no. 4, pp. 5–14.

Harrison, J. 1993, 'Spirituality and nursing practice', *Journal of Clinical Nursing*, vol. 2, pp. 211–17.

Highfield, M. 1992, 'Spiritual health of oncology patients: Nurses and patient perspectives', *Cancer Nursing*, vol. 15, no. 1, pp. 1–8.

Hodder, P. & Turley, A. (eds) 1989, *The Creative Option of Palliative Care*, Melbourne City Mission, Melbourne.

James, N. & Field, D. 1992, 'The routinization of hospice: Charisma and bureaucratization', *Social Science and Medicine*, vol. 34, no. 12, pp. 1363–75.

Kaczorowski, J. 1989, 'Spiritual wellbeing and anxiety in adults diagnosed with cancer', *Hospice Journal*, vol. 5, no. 3/4, pp. 105–16.

Kaye, R. & Robinson, K. 1994, 'Care-givers', *Image, Journal of Nursing Scholarship*, vol. 26, no. 3, pp. 218–21.

Kazanjian, M. 1997, 'The spiritual and psychological explanations for loss experience', *Hospice Journal*, vol. 12, no. 1, pp. 17–27.

Kirschling, J. & Pittman, J. F. 1989, 'Measurement of spiritual wellbeing: A hospice caregiver sample', *Hospice Journal*, vol. 5, no. 2, pp. 1–10.

Koenig, H. G. et al. 1999, Letter to the editor, *Scientific Review of Alternative Medicine*, vol. 3, p. 1.

Kuhn, T. 1970, *The Structure of Scientific Revolutions*, University of Chicago Press, Chicago.

Lamers, W. 1988, 'Hospice research: Some reflections', *Hospice Journal*, vol. 4, no. 3, pp. 3–11.

Little, M. 1995, *Humane Medicine*, Cambridge University Press, Cambridge.

Maddocks, I. 1990, 'Current concepts in palliative care', *Medical Journal of Australia*, vol. 152, pp. 535–9.

Mahoney, M. & Graci, G. 1999, 'The meanings and correlates of spirituality: Suggestions from an exploratory survey of experts', *Death Studies*, vol. 23, pp. 521–8.

McGrath, P. 1997a, 'Putting spirituality on the agenda: Hospice research findings on the "ignored" dimension', *Hospice Journal*, vol. 12, no. 4, pp. 269–71.

—— 1997b, 'Spirituality and discourse: A postmodern approach to hospice research', *Australian Health Review*, vol. 20, no. 2, pp. 116–28.

—— 1998a, 'A spiritual response to the challenge of routinization: A dialogue of discourses in a Buddhist-initiated hospice', *Qualitative Health Research*, vol. 8, no. 6, pp. 801–12.

—— 1998b, 'Buddhist spirituality—A compassionate perspective on hospice care', *Mortality*, vol. 3, no. 3, pp. 251–63.

—— 1998c, *A Question of Choice: Bioethical Reflections on a Spiritual Response to the Technological Imperative*, Ashgate Publishing, Hampshire.

—— 1999, 'Exploring spirituality through research: An important but challenging task', *Progress in Palliative Care*, vol. 7, no. 1, pp. 3–9.

—— & Newell, C. 2001, 'Insights on spirituality and serious illness from a patient's perspective', *Interface*, vol. 4, no. 2, pp. 101–9.

McNeill, P. 1993, *The Ethics and Politics of Human Experimentation*, Cambridge University Press, Cambridge.

—— 1998, 'Reason and emotion in medical ethics: A missing element', in *The Tasks of Medicine*, MacLennan & Petty, Sydney.

Meraviglia, M. 1999, 'Critical analysis of spirituality and its empirical indicators', *Journal of Holistic Nursing*, vol. 17, no. 1, pp. 18–33.

Messenger, R. & Roberts, K. 1994, 'The terminally ill: Serenity nursing interventions for hospice clients', *Journal of Gerontological Nursing*, vol. 20, no. 11, pp. 17–22.

Mickley, J. et al. 1998, 'God and the search for meaning among hospice care-givers', *Hospice Journal*, vol. 13, no. 4, pp. 1–17.

Millison, M. 1995, 'A review of the research on spiritual care and hospice', *Hospice Journal*, vol. 10, no. 4, pp. 3–18.

—— & Dudley, J. 1992, 'Providing spiritual support: A job for all hospice professionals', *Hospice Journal*, vol. 8, no. 4, pp. 49–66.

Mountain, D. & Muir, W. 2000, 'Spiritual wellbeing in psychiatric patients', *Irish Journal of Psychiatric Medicine*, vol. 17, no. 4, pp. 123–7.

Munley, A. 1983, *The Hospice Alternative; A New Context for Death and Dying*, Basic Books, New York.

Murray, R. & Zentner, J. 1985, *Nursing Concepts for Health Promotion*, Prentice Hall, Englewood Cliffs, New Jersey.

Nagai-Jacobson, M. & Burkhardt, M. 1989, 'Spirituality: Cornerstone of holistic nursing practice', *Holistic Nursing Practice*, vol. 1, no. 1, pp. 78–84.

Narayanasamy, A. 1993, 'Nurses' awareness and educational preparation in meeting their patients' spiritual needs', *Nurse Education Today*, vol. 13, no. 3, pp. 196–201.

O'Connell, L. 1996, 'Changing the culture of dying', *Health Services Administration*, vol. 77, no. 6, pp. 16–20.

O'Connor, P. 1988, 'The role of spiritual care in hospice', *American Journal of Hospice Care*, vol. 5, no. 2, pp. 31–7.

—— et al. 1997, 'Making the most and making sense: Ethnographic research on spirituality in palliative care', *Journal of Pastoral Care*, vol. 51, no. 1, pp. 25–36.

Oldnall, A. 1996, 'A critical analysis of nursing: Meeting the spiritual needs of patients', *Journal of Advanced Nursing*, vol. 23, pp. 138–44.

Pace, J. & Stables, J. 1997, 'Correlates of spiritual wellbeing in terminally ill patients with AIDS and terminally ill patients with cancer', *Journal of the Association of Nurses in AIDS Care*, vol. 8, no. 6, pp. 31–42.

Reed, P. 1987, 'Spirituality and wellbeing in terminally ill hospitalised adults', *Research in Nursing and Health*, vol. 10, pp. 335–344.

Reese, D. & Brown, D. 1997, 'Psychosocial and spiritual care in hospice: Differences between nursing, social work and clergy', *Hospice Journal*, vol. 12, no. 1, pp. 29–41.

Ross, L. 1994, 'Spiritual aspects of nursing', *Journal of Advanced Nursing*, vol. 19, pp. 439–47.

Saunders, C. 1981, 'The founding philosophy', in C. Saunders, D. Summers, & N. Teller (eds), *Hospice: The Living Idea*, Edward Arnold, London.

—— 1994, 'The dying patient', in R. Gillon (ed.), *Principles of Health Care Ethics*, John Wiley & Sons, Chichester.

Saynor, J. 1988, 'Existential and spiritual concerns of people with AIDS', *Journal of Palliative Care*, vol. 4, no. 4, pp. 61–5.

Sherman, D. 1996, 'Nurses' willingness to care for AIDS patients and spirituality, social support and death anxiety', *Image: Journal of Nursing Scholarship*, vol. 28, no. 3, pp. 205–13.

Siebold, C. 1992, *The Hospice Movement: Easing Death's Pains*, Twayne, New York.

Sims, C. 1987, 'Spiritual care as a part of holistic nursing', *Imprint*, vol. 34, pp. 663–5.

Smith, E. et al. 1993, 'Spiritual awareness, personal perspective on death, and psychosocial distress among cancer patients: An initial investigation', *Journal of Psychosocial Oncology*, vol. 11, no. 3, pp. 89–103.

Soeken, K. & Carson, V. 1986, 'Study measures nurses' attitudes about providing spiritual care', *Health Progress*, April, pp. 52–5.

—— 1987, 'Responding to the spiritual needs of the chronically ill', *Nursing Clinics of North America*, vol. 22, pp. 603–11.

Stepnick, A. & Perry, T. 1992, 'Preventing spiritual distress in the dying patient', *Journal of Psychosocial Nursing*, vol. 30, no. 1, pp. 17–24.

Stiles, M. 1990, 'The shining stranger: Nurse-family spiritual relationship', *Cancer Nursing*, vol. 13, no. 4, pp. 235–45.

Swinney, J. et al. 2001, 'Community assessment: A church community and the parish nurse', *Public Health Nursing*, vol. 18, no. 1, pp. 40–4.

Taylor, B. et al. 1997, 'Palliative nurses' perceptions of the nature and effect of their work', *International Journal of Palliative Nursing*, vol. 3, no. 5, pp. 253–8.

Taylor, E., Amenta, M., & Highfield, M. 1995, 'Spiritual care practices of oncology nurses', *Oncology Nursing Forum*, vol. 22, no. 1, pp. 31–9.

Wald, F., Foster, Z., & Wald, H. 1980, 'The hospice movement as a health care reform', *Nursing Outlook*, March, pp. 173–8.

Walter, T. 1997, 'The ideology and organization of spiritual care: Three approaches', *Palliative Medicine*, vol. 11, no. 1, pp. 21–30.

Walton, J. 1999, 'Spirituality of patients recovering from an acute myocardial infarction', *Journal of Holistic Nursing*, vol. 17, no. 1, pp. 34–53.

Weiner, E. et al. 2001, 'A qualitative study of physicians' own wellness promotion practices', *Western Journal of Medicine*, vol. 174, no. 1, pp. 19–24.

White, G. 2000, 'An inquiry into the concepts of spirituality and spiritual care', *International Journal of Palliative Nursing*, vol. 6, no. 10, pp. 479–84.

Woods, T. & Ironson, G. 1999, 'Religion and spirituality in the face of illness', *Journal of Health Psychology*, vol. 4, no. 3, pp. 393–412.

13

Dying as a Spiritual Quest

Bruce Rumbold

So many people demand answers that can't be refuted—not realising this is impossible if the issue is a transcendent one—when the search itself remains the important part.

Patrick White

The concept of dying as a quest appears in both traditional and contemporary discussions of death, although of course the nature and purpose of that quest may vary enormously. Some of the preceding chapters have already illustrated differences among religious understandings, while other contributors point to further variations in people's responses to experiencing life-threatening illness. Despite these variations, however, the quest portrayals agree that there are human possibilities inherent in encountering death, whether this be through contemplating our mortality or experiencing our dying. Some emphasise death as a gateway to another life, others the way knowledge of our finitude can revitalise our participation in life. Both forms are frequently framed as spiritual quests for a good death.

Dennis Klass remarks that '[p]erhaps all who set out on a spiritual quest do so of necessity. Surely a theme echoing through the spiritual literature of all religions is that a spiritual journey begins with a call that must be answered' (Klass 1999, p. 10). Today that call is frequently issued through an encounter with mortality, our own or another's, even though the call may not be heard until relatively late in life, for our society conspires to keep death at the margins of our awareness. In traditional societies it was religion that functioned both to keep mortality before people's gaze and to offer them the means to bear the knowledge of their finitude.

In traditional European societies, consciousness centred on human insufficiency in the face of finitude and death. This situation was remedied by religion, which provided an antidote to ontological anxiety through rituals and beliefs that preserved the soul, although not the body (Kolakowski 1982). Society's quest to transcend the fear of death was spearheaded by those who lived exemplary spiritual lives, the members of monastic communities, who laboured not only on their own account but also for the souls of districts in which their religious houses were situated. Thus life in this world was understood as preparation for life in a world to come. Death was the gateway to that new life, although it was also a moment of truth in which dying people might retard or advance their cause through the very manner of their dying (Clebsch & Jaekle 1967, pp. 178-189). The good death was one in which a dying person was able to reaffirm the central tenets of belief and claim his or her place in the church, whose influence held not only in this world but also in the next. Death, while a barrier, was not totally impermeable to the living for, through the church, interventions could be made to aid friends and family members in their postmortem journey.

Death could not be ignored in traditional European society—it was too much a part of everyday experience—but as the Middle Ages drew to a close a sense of the nearness of death was increasingly fostered by the church in order to maintain its social dominance (Bauman 1998). The heightened awareness—even obsession—with death in the late Middle Ages led to a situation where the demands of piety simply became impossible for people who had to carry on a normal life in society (Delumeau 1990). This dilemma was the soil from which the Reformation arose. Protestantism began as a movement of popular piety that wrested responsibility for spiritual life from the church and returned it to individuals. Rather than relying upon participation in socially agreed, church-authorised rituals to achieve salvation, individuals now became responsible for their decision to affiliate with one of the various religious movements that arose as church authority fragmented. The communal quest by which the church mediated between the living and the dead was replaced by quests in which individuals were responsible through their conscience to God. One implication of Protestantism's rejection of the church's mediating role was to remove the connection between the eternal destiny of the departed and their living kin. No longer could the living work on behalf of the dead. The last days and hours of life became a time in which the dying witnessed to the faith by which they had lived and so encouraged and supported those left behind. Dying was the culmination of the individual's spiritual quest, albeit a quest carried out in a particular community and witnessed by members of that community.

Death continued to be a focus for spiritual reflection, and human insufficiency remained the subject for religious remedies, well into the modern era. Dying continued to be understood as embarkation on another life, and the care offered to dying people by family and local community was designed to aid that transition, to prepare the person for what he or she would become. The responsibilities of the dying person and those who offered care were well understood (Rumbold 1986, pp. 80–3). Indeed, they were well rehearsed, for the anticipation of death was a major focus for reflection and spiritual growth. Thus the great Evangelical divine, William Law (1728, 1965, p. 243ff), recommends for each day's evening prayer that

> The subject ... most proper ... at that time is death. Let your prayers, therefore, then be wholly upon it, reckoning upon all the dangers, uncertainties and terrors of death; let them contain everything that can affect and awaken your mind into just apprehensions of it. Let your petitions be all for right sentiments of the approach and importance of death; and beg of God, that your mind may be possessed with such a sense of its nearness, that you may have it always in your thoughts, do everything as in sight of it, and make every day a preparation for it.
>
> And then commit yourself to sleep, as into the hands of God; as one that is to have no more opportunities of doing good; but is to awake among spirits that are separate from the body, and awaiting for the judgement of the last great day.

Life was to be lived courageously in the presence of death. Christians were to participate in life as fully as they could, while at the same time always being prepared to relinquish their place to others. Death was a gift that injected significance into the present while putting dreams into perspective and puncturing inflated views of oneself.

A major transition took place during the nineteenth century as religious authority concerning death was replaced with that of the new scientific medicine. In the closing decades of the eighteenth century, some physicians had begun to involve themselves in the emerging science of pathological anatomy. Death, hitherto a barrier to medical knowledge because it ended communication with the patient, became instead the gateway to new knowledge gained through dissection of corpses. This proved to be merely the first move in an alliance between medicine and the sciences that was reshaping Western worldviews and led in due course to a new form of medical practice (Foucault 1973). As scientific thinking and knowledge gained in influence, so too did the new medicine. Deathbed accounts in the nineteenth century show a gradual shift from religious to medical authority. At the beginning of this period religious interventions were primary, with comfort seen as secondary to making a good death. By the end of the century some medical practitioners would, in the name of the patient's comfort, turn away a clergyman bringing the Eucharist (Jalland 1997). The individual's quest in dying became increasingly subject to medical direction.

For most of the twentieth century, death was treated primarily as a medical event. It was not, however, welcomed as an area of medical expertise so much as reluctantly accepted as an outcome of unsuccessful treatment. The medical quest concerning dying was focused on avoiding or delaying death. There was silence when death became inevitable. Correspondingly, discussions of death and dying as part of human experience disappeared within the society at large. Whether a death could be called good or not was a private matter. In public—at least in times of peace—death was good if it was attended by technically correct medical procedures (Kastenbaum 1975) and accomplished with minimum disruption. While early in the century attempts were made to develop scientific approaches to traditional issues of quest such as survival and afterlife, these were given short shrift by the religious and the scientific authorities (Irwin 2000). As the church lost its earlier dominance over death, deferring instead to medicine, both death and eternal life also drifted gradually to the margins of Christian consciousness. Within the Christian tradition voices such as those of William Law or the hymn writers who constantly reminded us that our experiences and insights are framed and limited by human mortality disappeared. They have been replaced in contemporary religious practice by voices that speak largely of this-worldly feelings and, occasionally, of other-worldly hopes, but seldom of how these feelings and hopes might be grounded in our living and dying, and never of how we might best make the transition from one world to the next, 'make a good death' as Christian tradition would call it.

Now, once again, the situation is changing and the medicalisation of death is under review. The major evidence of change is renewed discussion of dying as a human quest. Death as a medical problem is tempered by renewed investigation of death as human possibility. Some of this discussion began within medicine itself, with the emergence of the hospice movement in the 1960s (Clark 1998). Hospice care revived traditional models of a good death in a way that was informed, but not determined, by modern medical practice (Walter 1994). It intentionally placed itself at the margins of the health system, drawing instead upon the support of local communities in order to claim the freedom to develop new forms of holistic care that it hoped would in due course permeate the rest of the health system. In the words of Dame Cicely Saunders, founder of the hospice movement, 'We moved out [of the National Health Service] so that attitudes and knowledge could move back in' (Saunders et al. 1981, p. 4). However, the hospice movement has in its more recent guise of palliative care been drawn increasingly back into the mainstream; indeed, it has actively sought the mainstream to increase access and ensure continuing funding (Hockley 1997), although with rather different results to those envisaged by Saunders. The good death of palliative care emerges from the cooperative efforts of the dying person, family, and caring team, which requires an egalitarianism the health system finds hard to accommodate. Palliative care is currently at risk of being conformed to a clinical model in which the social and spiritual dimensions of care are at best marginal or optional, even though attention to these dimensions was what distinguished the hospice movement in the first place (Rumbold 1998).

Other contemporary ideas of a good death are also emerging, including the proposal that medical practitioners should be permitted, even required, to assist patients to die should they be able to demonstrate and defend their desire to do so. Euthanasia is one logical outcome of a customer-centred approach to healthcare delivery. Yet another is the idea of a 'natural death', which attempts to return agency to the dying person by minimising the influence of medical interventions, thereby sounding at times more like a way back to the past than a way forward into the future. In recent debates these differing ideas of a good death have been presented as competitors, although each draws attention to elements lacking in many contemporary deaths: informed cooperation between carers and those for whom they care, maintenance of a sense of personal agency for dying people, and refusal to let the search for medical treatment become the dominant story of people's last days.

QUESTING AND DYING

What then are the stories that emerge when life and death meet in conversation and contestation as they do in life-threatening illness? Arthur Frank, himself a survivor of both cardiac disease and cancer, suggests that contemporary illness narratives are found in three basic forms: restitution narratives, chaos narratives, and quest narratives (Frank 1995). These categories have already been introduced in chapter 5, but are reviewed here for the sake of this account.

Restitution narratives

In these stories sickness is an aberration that should be overcome for life to retain its meaning. Yesterday I was healthy, today I'm sick, but tomorrow I'll be well again. The experience of illness is an interruption to the overall story of life, and the future that beckons is remarkably like the (romanticised) past.

This story dominates medical institutions, cancer support groups, and society in general. Suffering becomes a problem to be solved by the experts. Thus this is a story about the triumph of medicine; only by default is it the teller's story. To adopt it as my story I must invest my identity in someone else's narrative (in essence take on Parsons's sick role). To resist is costly, too. Costain Schou and Hewison (1999) describe how the demands of illness and treatment dominate the personal and life agendas of people with cancer, forcing relinquishment of important aspects of identity and focusing identity in their new role as a patient. The absence of alternatives is even more marked for other forms of life-threatening illness where disclosure of prognosis is less overt (Field 1996).

Restitution narratives are stories about recovery, preferably about cure. They can, however, carry us through dying if we adopt the approach that, while recovery may no longer be a possibility for us, our actions may contribute to the restitution of others.

Chaos narratives

In its purest form chaos lacks a storyline. We hear instead fragments of stories from people who are stuck in an unbearable present without meaningful access to past or present. They lack a voice because it appears that no one is in control, no coherent story can be told because the suffering is too great.

Paradoxically, the chaos and the suffering must be acknowledged if anything is to change. Chaos is their truth at the moment. But too often a restitution story is immediately imposed: sufferers are declared depressed and their suffering treated as a clinical symptom, a problem to be solved rather than a mystery to be encountered.

Quest narratives

Unlike the two previous forms, the teller owns this narrative. The restitution and chaos narratives are both there in the background: I would suggest that they are necessary preludes to the transformation involved in the quest narrative. The teller refuses to have his or her story narrowed to an expert's preferred narrative, endures the deconstruction that takes place in chaos, and seeks a new integration of previous narratives with possibilities that arise in the changed circumstances.

A quest narrative constructs illness as a journey—neither an aberration nor a dead end. It is a journey that begins with a call to leave the safety of the known and journey into the unknown experiences of serious illness. Responding to the call involves initiation into suffering and trial, then (hopefully), transformation, and return. The one who perseveres finds a way. Restitution narratives are resisted as too easy or too inadequate a story, while chaos is held at bay by the teller's courage and sense of identity and integrity.

Most illness stories published today are quest narratives, like classic religious narratives. This is not surprising. A major strand in most religions is the use of stories for teaching so that, for example, stories of the saints recall exemplary lives that serve as a model for all. The new illness stories serve a similar purpose. They are narratives which, almost without exception, demonstrate exemplary responses to illness—a determination to survive, the importance of individual will and control, the significance of personal supports. It is for this reason that Frank asserts that those on quest bear testimony to experiences and knowledge that challenge current schema. He uses the word 'witness' rather than 'survivor' for this reason—the people who go on quest produce stories that open up new frontiers for others who will listen to their tale. As they testify to the experiences of their journeys, they witness to new possibilities for the human spirit. Such testimony of course is not limited to survivors, but may continue in the witness of those who have shared a person's quest and witnessed that person's death.

The growing body of testimony—much of it in popular and alternative literatures or at the fringes of academic enquiry—is a major resource for spiritual care. It shapes media interests and invites others to make their own explorations of illness, encouraging them to find possibilities in overcoming illness or in living their dying (Weenolsen 1996). It draws attention to the fact that mere survival is not enough and that many of those who are successful according to the values of a restitution narrative find themselves cured but dislocated, unable to return to their former lives.

While traditional religious accounts and contemporary illness narratives have a common interest in the spiritual possibilities inherent in actively engaging illness and death, they also differ in some fundamental respects. Religious narratives point beyond the self to the ultimate meaning uncovered on the quest, while contemporary accounts focus more upon the experiences along the way, a shift in focus that was discussed in chapter 1. It reflects a change in consciousness brought about by modernity. Religious experience, once its own interpreter, has become interpretable by the natural sciences, psychology in particular. Thus Maslow could suggest that 'organised religion can be thought of as an effort to communicate peak-experiences to non-peakers' (Maslow 1964, p. 24). Similar interpretations now dominate contemporary quests, which seek experiences more than look for fresh ways of understanding the world. Their concern is now for self-identity, not remedies for self-insufficiency, uncertainty is no longer about ontological matters so much as uncertainty about identity. Traditional spiritual disciplines are often invoked, but in new ways. For example meditation, which originated as a discipline for losing the self, is now employed for finding or preserving self-identity. Thus while traditional mysticism spoke of losing oneself in the divine, the new spiritualities talk about finding the divine within oneself (Chopra 1999, p. 202). 'What distinguishes the postmodern strategy of peak-experience from one promoted by religions, is that far from celebrating the assumed human insufficiency and weakness, it appeals to the full development of human inner psychological and bodily resources and presumes infinite human potency' (Bauman 1998, p. 70). Transcendence becomes this-worldly as much as—or instead of—other-worldly.

Despite these changes, quest continues to be a useful metaphor to describe people's search for possibilities in their dying. Sometimes the quest is initiated as people are confronted with their mortality through their own illness, or the illness or death of another. Sometimes an existing quest is challenged and focused through the encounter with illness and death, as Maggie May's account in chapter 6 illustrates. At times the challenge will bring about a change of direction. Some who have previously sought experiences will find themselves seeking understanding; while some who previously have sought understanding will find they lack confirmatory experience. Again, the issue of spiritual practice becomes important, including access to a community of practice that is flexible enough to offer a range of spiritual paths. The deregulation of religion and the opening up of alternative spiritual resources provides rich—if at times confusing—resources for developing spiritual quests in dying.

The shift in consciousness that has opened up these resources nevertheless creates its own problems.

> If the religious version of peak-experience was used to reconcile the faithful to a life of misery and hardship, the postmodern version reconciles its followers to life organised around the duty of an avid, perpetual, though never definitely gratifying consumption ... The axiom which underpins all [self-improvement] movements is that experiencing, like all other human faculties, is above all a *technical* problem, and that acquiring the capacity for it is a matter of mastering the appropriate *techniques* (Bauman 1998, pp. 70–1).

Spiritual disciplines that become techniques—an end in themselves—are not able to effect the formation of a mature self. Spiritual guides who employ disciplines as techniques are unlikely to offer the sort of relationship in which genuine care, and hence spiritual transformation, can take place.

FACILITATING QUEST

Traditionally, spiritual care has involved supporting another's quest for meaning, or wholeness, or transcendence. It has depended upon known pathways, established disciplines, by which the spiritual guide could instruct and support others on their journeys. The goal of the journey was a new postmortem identity, preceded by a death that relied upon and validated a lifetime of practice.

This disciplined, staged approach to spiritual growth permitted, in fact encouraged, spiritual diagnosis which guided spiritual care. The distinctive feature of this diagnosis was that it was carried out by mutual participation in a shared framework of understanding. Experiences at particular points on the journey were identified and interpreted according to an overall story, which had been prepared on the basis of reports of previous travellers. Diagnosis linked current experience with the overarching story. The guide was a companion on the same road rather than an expert on the topography of the spiritual realm.

These dynamics still hold. Because spirituality describes the way we make our lives, there are times we need another to discern what indeed characterises our spirituality. For we live within it, we do not construct or control it. We may be aware of ways in which we support our spirituality, but we cannot completely control or direct it. We find that spirituality is about connectedness, but also about incompleteness. It is about knowledge, but equally about what we do not know. It is about coherence and integrity, but also about vulnerability. It is about belief, but equally about doubt.

In the face of change or crisis—and dying can face us with both—we may find ourselves needing to explore roads not taken. Thus, those whose spirituality has to this point taken the form of dwelling, may need to seek, while those who have sought may discover also a need to dwell (see chapter 1 for discussion of these forms). While these transitions need not take place in a religious framework, particularly an institutional religious framework, it is nevertheless significant that the great religious traditions have always maintained within themselves the tensions between dwelling and seeking, knowledge and doubt, presence and absence.

Dying needs to be connected with life, not death. Even while dying we are looking at death from the standpoint of the living, albeit as a person who will soon enter the experience of death. According to many traditional religious views a spirituality disconnected from the rest of life is no spirituality at all. Embeddedness in the everyday is a mark of authentic spirituality.

SPIRITUAL CARE AND PALLIATIVE CARE

The genius of the hospice vision was the way it blurred boundaries that characterised the healthcare system of its day. It challenged the lack of personal involvement in professional care, insisting that to care for someone also required caring about them. It insisted that spiritual care was not merely a matter of permitting the private religious practices of some patients, but that these practices should be integrated with other aspects of care for all participants in the program, whether or not they were formally religious.

Palliative care's reconnection of the hospice vision with mainstream healthcare has led to a situation where palliative care programs struggle to develop ways of offering spiritual care in contexts that are increasingly clinically organised. Such contexts may be admirably suited for the purposes of delivering short-term physical care, but the environments and strategies that are effective for such physical or psychological care may be less than effective or even harmful if extended to other dimensions of care.

Palliative care programs usually have designated pastoral care as the discipline with a holding brief for spiritual care in much the same way that psychologists provide a focus for the palliative care team's psychological care and social workers usually take primary responsibility for devising and delivering social interventions. In the discussion that follows I will explore issues in offering spiritual care assuming the involvement within the team of a pastoral care worker as the person who takes particular responsibility for spiritual care. I will also assume that the worker is formed in the pastoral care tradition that espouses a social—or holistic—model of care, despite the fact that many contemporary pastoral care practitioners have (usually unintentionally) compromised or neglected the social dimensions of their tradition in using individualistic counselling methods as the major tool of their practice.

The social model of care that informs pastoral care sets up some significant tensions with a clinical approach. For example:

• The pastoral tradition supports a complex and diverse understanding of human needs and responses; clinical perceptions tend to be simple and categorical.

• The pastoral tradition emphasises that spiritual insight might be achieved through relationships characterised by mutual participation and vulnerability; clinical interest tends to be in objective assessments conducted by expert professionals.

• The pastoral tradition understands that care relies upon and creates community; clinical approaches to care separate sick individuals from the well community, replacing wider social roles with the role of patient.

Palliative care at its best seeks to maintain these differing perceptions in creative tension. When it resolves the tension it tends to do so in favour of a clinical approach, but this marginalises—and to an extent compromises—social and spiritual aspects of care, as Allan Kellehear indicates in chapter 11.

In order to focus this discussion further I will explore some of the implications of practising spiritual care according to the standards promoted by the umbrella body for Australian palliative care programs, Palliative Care Australia (1999). These standards identify six domains of palliative care practice.

Standards for palliative care provision
Palliative Care Australia, 3rd edn, October 1999

DOMAIN 1	PHYSICAL
DOMAIN 2	PSYCHOLOGICAL
DOMAIN 3	SOCIAL
DOMAIN 4	SPIRITUAL
DOMAIN 5	CULTURAL
DOMAIN 6	STRUCTURAL

Each domain contains between one and five standards. For the spiritual domain these are as follows.

4.1 The spiritual dimensions of the patient and family are acknowledged, explored, and responded to appropriately.

4.2 The religious beliefs of the patient and family are recognised and respected.

4.3 Appropriate spiritual and religious support for patients, families and carers is provided.

Each standard has attached to it a number of criteria by which its practice may be verified. For the spiritual care standards, these criteria are as follows.

4.1 The spiritual dimensions of the patient and family are acknowledged, explored, and responded to appropriately.
Criteria
1 A spiritual assessment process or validated tool is used to identify the spiritual strengths and needs of the patient and family.
2 A care plan, based on the spiritual assessment and reflecting the patient's right to self-determination is developed and documented.
3 The care plan reflects an acknowledgement of the spiritual dimension and provides opportunity for its expression.
4 Access to spiritual awareness development programs is facilitated for staff and volunteers.

4.2 The religious beliefs of the patient and family are recognised and respected.
Criteria
1 The service displays sensitivity in its use of religious symbols and icons.
2 The patient and family is encouraged to display the religious symbols and icons of their belief systems.
3 Opportunities for the patient and family to conduct rites or practise spiritual rituals are facilitated by the palliative care service.
4 Staff and volunteer development programs build an awareness of diverse religious beliefs and traditions.

4.3 Appropriate spiritual and religious support for patients, families, and carers is provided.
Criteria
1 The interdisciplinary team will include appropriately trained and funded pastoral care professionals.

2   A structured and documented process for accessing pastoral care is in evidence.

3   A directory of pastoral care resources is available.

4   The pastoral care service, on behalf of patients and families, facilitates appropriate contacts with community based religious or spiritual support groups or individuals.

The criteria are based upon the understanding that spiritual care practice is as much about creating an environment for spiritual nurture as it is offering particular services. Obviously, meeting the criteria requires a wide range of knowledge and skills. It is still assumed that these skills will be provided— or at least coordinated—by pastoral care workers, but the job description of such a pastoral care worker goes well beyond the traditional chaplaincy role. Drawing on these criteria as well as upon chaplaincy standards as drafted by, for example, the Australian Health and Welfare Chaplains' Association (1998), we can develop a description of pastoral care practice.

KEY ROLES OF A PASTORAL CARE WORKER

- Identify and assess spiritual strengths and needs of patients and families.
- Participate as a member of the interdisciplinary team in devising comprehensive care plans that include strategies for spiritual care.
- Prepare, lead, or facilitate religious and spiritual rituals as required.
- Provide pastoral counselling and spiritual direction.
- Provide information on ethical, religious, and pastoral matters.
- Develop a directory of pastoral care resources.
- Coordinate involvement of community-based religious and spiritual care providers.
- Coordinate access to spiritual awareness development programs for staff and volunteers.
- Provide pastoral care training as required.
- Supervise pastoral care contributions of other staff and volunteer helpers.

Knowledge required

- Religious and spiritual traditions.
- Principles of healthcare and palliative care.

- Cultural perspectives (including contemporary culture) on spirituality, health, and illness.
- Interpersonal processes.
- Knowledge of self.

Skills required

- Listening.
- Counselling.
- Spiritual direction.
- Training and educating.
- Designing and leading ritual.
- Recording and reporting.
- Liaising with colleagues and community groups.

To discuss in detail the various facets of this description would be a task for a monograph, not a chapter. Further resources for many of the tasks identified here may be found in Irion (1988) and Cobb (2001). I want to explore in the remainder of this chapter issues raised by the requirement to assess spiritual strengths and needs, and some of the implications for the training of pastoral care workers and other health professionals. I will conclude with some further observations on the knowledge and skills required for offering spiritual care.

ASSESSING SPIRITUAL NEED

The approach to spiritual care described, discussed, or implied by the various contributors to this collection is consultative, discursive, grounded in genuine relationship, and open to possibility. It may draw upon, but will not be dictated to or confined by, particular religious, social, or cultural traditions. We assume that spiritual care aims at creating an environment in which people are supported and encouraged to look beyond the problems they encounter to find creative ways of solving, absorbing or transcending them. Thus spiritual care begins with relationships in which people feel safe to explore the issues of deepest concern to them. It continues as those who offer care provide personal support, information, resources, ideas, and referrals appropriate to the exploration initiated within the relationship.

In the light of this, any assessment of spiritual strengths and needs (first criterion, Standard 4.1 above) should begin with careful and respectful description, preferably a description developed in consultation with, and validated by, the person who is the subject of the description. The description may include a statement of strengths and needs if the person so desires, but the major focus should be the support the person requires to remain responsible for his or her own spiritual quest. It is important to clarify the extent to which a spiritual assessment is disclosed to the caring team. Information made available in a genuine, mutual relationship is privileged communication; it should not be disclosed within the team without permission. Nor can it be assumed that someone else can pick up the conversation at the point another team member has left it. Conversations about spiritual matters require trusting relationships. Team members have no right to expect spiritual (or emotional) disclosures from their clients; their responsibility is to offer the sort of relationship in which disclosure might be possible. All too often a client's silence under emotional or spiritual probing is labelled 'denial' by some practitioners. It might be better to assume that clients are unwilling to expose their concerns to practitioners who indulge in such labelling behaviours.

In this understanding, spiritual care begins with particular sorts of relationships, is concerned with good process more than specific outcomes, and attends to possibilities more than to solving problems that may be perceived. It refuses to take agency away from the client, and endeavours to restore that agency if it has been eroded by other approaches to care. This stands in tension with many of the spiritual assessment tools that have been developed or published in recent years. Most of these use an itemised survey approach that seems more concerned with labelling emotions and identifying problems than with developing possibilities, reflecting the clinical disciplines from which such approaches arise. These assessments endeavour to assess risk through observation or diagnostic questioning that allows an observer or clinician to make a judgment of need and prescribe responses. From here it is only a short step to expecting spiritual care to justify itself by its ability to improve clinical outcomes and measures. In contrast to this, traditional spiritual care—and also the style of care advocated here—adopts a possibility-oriented approach focused on the testimony of the client. 'Where is there life, or energy, for you in this situation?' 'What gives you hope?' 'What is your prayer?' 'To whom do you belong?' are the core questions of traditional spiritual direction and could well continue to be the focus of interest for today's spiritual care practitioners.

Fundamentally, an itemised survey approach fails to take account of the dynamic nature of spirit or the ambiguity of observation. What I choose to disclose under surveillance will differ—often markedly—from what I might choose to disclose to a companion, friend, or mentor. A surveillance approach, such as a survey, may also on occasion open up issues that the interviewer either fails to recognise or is not competent to deal with (Cobb 1998). In the light of such strategies Walter is right to ask whether 'spiritual care can be organised on a large scale and still be worthy of the name' (Walter 1997, p. 30).

Our contention here is that spiritual care can be organised, but not according to a clinical model that endeavours to set up routines to be carried out irrespective of the practitioner (or the patient) involved. What can be organised is a systematic assessment of the resources available to the person, and respectful, consultative discussion that may lead to developing a spiritual care plan. One of the results of such a discussion could, of course, be agreement that a patient should not be expected to address spiritual issues with members of the palliative care team. The outcome of spiritual care should be chosen by the client, although the process of offering spiritual care should be made accountable.

A practical dilemma confronts pastoral care workers in programs that already favour the use of validated tools or itemised assessment schedules. It is to be hoped that workers will use these tools or schedules as a basis for discussion with patients, thus developing collaborative relationships rather than replacing them with a task, in much the same way that Fischer advocates individualising psychological assessment tools (Fischer 1985).

TRAINING IN SPIRITUAL CARE

To date, much of the training provided for spiritual care has been either informational or inspirational, lacking in both theory and process. This seems true of the training offered within tertiary vocational programs as well as the inservice opportunities provided by palliative care services.

Certainly, the pastoral care worker description above specifies access to a range of information, and the actual implementation of the tasks requires some creativity and inspiration. However, training as a pastoral care worker also needs to provide grounding in appropriate theory, including that of religious studies and public health as well as pastoral care itself, noting that all three as multidisciplinary areas have some methodologies in common, social science methodologies in particular. Training needs to develop the abilities of building theory for spirituality (Kellehear 2000) and of attending to personal, interpersonal, and organisational processes. To achieve this, training itself must be multidisciplinary so that students can develop skills by engaging different perspectives, not being encouraged by teachers to adopt a single disciplinary frame. The latter approach too often leads to the colonisation or capture of one worldview by another, usually the reduction of a complex, culturally informed approach to a set of simple (or simplistic) techniques.

Training in spiritual care must include a significant amount of experiential learning in order to develop workers who are reflective practitioners. As John Paver indicates in chapter 10, supervision is an essential aspect of this, to equip workers to develop insight into their own personal process and learn to take responsibility for their ongoing development. Because spiritual care is person centred, training in spiritual care must ensure that workers are aware of the differing perspectives out of which care may be provided. This is especially important for workers who are trained in both a clinical discipline and in pastoral care, lest spiritual care strategies from a person-centred approach be converted to techniques in clinically shaped practice. Real difficulties can arise because clinical training focuses upon identifying problems and providing solutions, while spiritual care training equips the worker to accompany others on a search, that is, it involves other modes of relating and other modes of knowing. The skill of working in another's framework comes even harder when your primary disciplinary formation is as a clinician, that is, one who can distinguish symptom from sign, illness from health, truth from error. It is of course important also that pastoral care workers trained within specific religious traditions are able to separate their own religious concerns from those of their clients. Again, this requires the sort of insight into practice that skilled supervision can provide.

More positively, formation in more than one discipline is of great benefit provided one approach does not dominate the other. The capacity to revise perspectives or reframe understandings that is gained from complementary training experiences can be a significant resource when helping others to explore fresh ways of connecting experiences or reframing life narratives.

OFFERING SPIRITUAL CARE

As the preceding discussion has indicated, the ability to offer spiritual care begins with the attitude and perceptions of care-givers and their openness to genuine human encounter (Montgomery 1991). Spiritual care-givers need the ability to wait, to tolerate (even welcome) ambiguity, to be vulnerable, and to attend to process more than outcome. These abilities are formed less by instruction than by reflective practice. Those who seek to offer spiritual care should demonstrate in themselves some of the qualities they hope to awaken in others. They are companions rather than instructors. Embodiment is more important than information.

Offering spiritual care requires discernment, as the ultimate welfare of a patient may not be served best by uncritical support of any or all spiritual ideas or practices. The emphasis on personal autonomy, control, and survival that permeates many contemporary spiritual care systems can foster spiritual-ities that deny death. These systems promote spiritual practices as survival strategies—place them in a restitution narrative, to use Frank's terminol-ogy—and use them to serve a predetermined goal of recovery from illness. Such practices may support a person for a while, but will prove inadequate if recovery does not eventuate. Then the task of the spiritual companion is to support the person in the ensuing chaos, perhaps offering some guidance on ways that existing spiritual practices can be liberated from a restitution narra-tive and employed in a quest. Spiritual practices may begin as techniques harnessed to a specific goal, but to become transformative they must be allowed to change us and open us to fresh possibility, including the possibil-ities inherent in our deepest reluctances and fears.

Effective spiritual care has to negotiate the tension between respect for the other, the patient, and the recognition that there are limits to the other's autonomy as death approaches. There may be times when respect involves challenging a perspective that is inadequate to the circumstances or a strategy that is no longer effective. Similarly, spiritual companions may need to nego-tiate tensions between accountability to the patient and accountability to an overall care plan, developing strategies for care while avoiding reducing spiri-tual disciplines to techniques that serve clinically determined goals. Practising spiritual care requires us to deal respectfully with difference, neither ignoring it nor seeking to remove it. Companions need resilience and the capacity to learn from the people they accompany (Drewery with McKenzie 1999).

Spiritual care practice aims at developing possibilities. Its focus is less upon the problems that life-threatening illness can bring than it is upon the life of the person. Spiritual care seeks to promote health, supporting people to develop, and expand their understanding of health so that life can be found even in the presence of death. A major dilemma for pastoral care workers in palliative care programs is that issues may be raised when it is too late to do anything much about them: patients are admitted to the program because physical symptoms require attention, but the appropriate time for intervention in social and spiritual domains is long past. An approach to spirituality that signals freedom to create your own truth may be experienced as yet another burden when time—and creative energy—is short.

Spiritual care emerges most naturally and easily in an environment that supports and encourages quest. In one sense health services are already such environments, except that their quest for health is normally narrowly interpreted as a quest for cure and it is the physician, not the patient, who does the questing.

Health, then, becomes no longer an option for those who cannot be restored to wellness. Health can, however, be viewed more broadly than this. Understanding health in participatory ways, understanding that health is created by people in communities, not an intrinsic commodity lost through the impact of illness or disease, means that people can continue to explore health and see themselves as healthy even while experiencing life-threatening illness (Kagawa-Singer 1993). It is vital for spiritual care that palliative care programs, in addition to their alliances with mainstream health services, continue alliances with holistic and public health associations that promote participatory, social models of health. Without this there is always the risk that spiritual care will be placed alongside (or at the margins of) other approaches to care, without taking proper cognisance of the way the spiritual emerges from within and among the range of human experience.

THE QUEST FOR HEALTH IN PALLIATIVE CARE

A health promoting approach to palliative care (Kellehear 1999) invites us to reconnect health and dying, thereby challenging the tendency to regard palliative care simply as an end-stage service and health as something that can no longer be promoted in the face of life-threatening illness. It asserts that awareness of dying should be made part of life, that social knowledge of the human experience of dying should be increased, so that public discussion of what constitutes a good death can move beyond simplistic assertions about whether euthanasia should be considered a patient's right or a doctor's offence. It suggests not that dying be removed from clinical attention, but that clinical care be seen as part of a broad social and cultural context in which each person's dying takes place.

Health promotion, which is grounded in the new public health (Baum 1998), has an understanding of health that correlates well with a pastoral approach to care. Missionary doctor turned pastoral care teacher, Michael Wilson, asserts that 'there is no way to health through the cure of illness … Rather than trying to reach health by understanding illness, we must first try to understand health, in the light of which we may be able to say something about being well or ill' (Wilson 1976, p. 55). Consistent with this, the new public health sees health as a quality that communities must achieve rather than something that appears when disease is absent. It is open to the complexity of human experience, including human experience of the divine.

If spiritual care can be framed as an integral aspect of the quest for health, this opens up much broader possibilities for spiritual interventions. While only a few practitioners may focus directly upon spiritual issues, and others do so on occasion, all healthcare practitioners can be involved in creating environments conducive to spiritual care. Such environments will no longer juxtapose living and dying, but will recognise dying as a part of living, a good death as something that is best prepared for by seeking to live fully for all of our days.

Much of the preceding discussion has been about how pastoral care workers can facilitate spiritual care, including a strong emphasis on the need for pastoral workers to avoid allowing spiritual care to revert to a clinical approach. So how might clinicians contribute to a good death? A starting point is the role that clinicians, medical practitioners in particular, continue to have as social custodians of dying and gatekeepers to services for the dying. The referrals doctors make can be crucial in a person's experience of illness; they should reflect a broadly social, not just a narrowly clinical, perspective. That is, doctors should refer out as well as refer in, pointing people to resources in their community as well as resources in the health services.

Referring people into the health system ensures that they receive state of the art treatment, but it does not ensure that they will receive what they need to make a good death. Travelling the route of secondary and tertiary health service referral can further fragment people's experience and confound their understandings. The complexity of treatment, the diversity of practitioners encountered, and the sheer time and effort involved, means that for many people treatment comes to dominate their lives (Costain Schou & Hewison 1999). The search for a cure becomes their source for meaning and they lose touch with the roles that have given them meaning in the past.

Further, the effect of pursuing treatment can be that the possibility of dying is discounted so long as there is some possibility of cure. People are then referred to palliative care programs after treatment options are exhausted and clinical problems are escalating. This is too late to make a positive difference to people's dying, for social and pastoral interventions need to be made well before disablement. People with a life-threatening illness deserve the opportunity to explore the possibilities of dying at the same time they are exploring the options for ongoing treatment. They need to be confirmed in their continuing social identities and encouraged to explore new or neglected aspects of their lives, not just substitute for all these their new role as a patient. Only when people are able to explore the resources of their own lives and of their communities can a search for cure become a search for healing, even if it turns out—as eventually it will for all of us—that the road to healing leads through death.

Supporting the search for healing involves referring out as well as referring in. In a different society there might be other gatekeepers to make such referrals, but in a society such as ours, where dying remains largely medicalised, it falls to clinicians to initiate the outward movement as well. I readily acknowledge that referring out is not as simple as referring in, in part because community networks are much more diffuse and often less accountable than are health service networks. It should, however, be possible to set up arrangements where a single referral to, say, a local community health service or congregational care agency links a patient to someone who will work with them to explore strategies for creating health in the midst of illness.

There is enormous support in people hearing each other's stories. Those of us who have ongoing contact with people with a life-threatening illness should encourage them to tell, write, or paint, their stories, even if the only listeners, readers, or viewers will be their families or friends. It is somewhat ironic that the accounts proclaiming the fullness of life discovered through facing death are nowadays found not in religious publications but in first-person accounts published in palliative care journals and popular magazines. There are stories about how the imminence of death has led to liberation that people have avoided in the rest of their lives. Stories about near-death experiences that have transformed the way people now live. Stories about encounters with angels who have redirected people's paths (and spawned the odd telemovie along the way). Stories you will find in the New Age section of your local bookshop, alongside a dwindling remnant of religious materials that also make their way there.

LOOKING AHEAD

Clearly, spirituality and spiritual care today are in a state of flux, a situation that offers significant opportunity for looking at health in fresh ways but also the danger that these signs of new directions will be subsumed within old paradigms of care. The new spiritual care is an invitation not only to personal reorientation, but to reorientation of health services and of society at large. A critical test will be whether the new spirituality can connect living and dying in ways that revitalise living. Traditional societies tended to discount living in comparison with a life to come after death, while modern society tended to ignore death, seeing it as the negation of living. Neither approach seems adequate today and, as a result, new understandings are emerging. Palliative care has played an important role in raising the issue of death and dying after a long period of public silence. To continue to make a contribution it needs now to take its stories of good deaths and courageous quests out into the community, opening up possibilities that invite us all to join in the quest.

REFERENCES

Australian Health and Welfare Chaplains' Association 1998, *Chaplaincy Standards*, unpublished draft.

Baum, F. 1998, *The New Public Health: An Australian Perspective*, Oxford University Press, Melbourne.

Bauman, Z. 1998, 'Postmodern religion', in Heelas, P. (ed.), *Religion, Modernity and Postmodernity*, Blackwell, Oxford, pp. 55–78.

Chopra, D. 1999, *Everyday Immortality: A Concise Course in Spiritual Transformation*, Harmony Books, New York.

Clark, D. 1998, 'Originating a movement: Cicely Saunders and the development of St Christopher's Hospice, 1957–67', *Mortality*, vol. 3, pp. 43–63.

Clebsch, R. & Jaekle, W. 1967, *Pastoral Care in Historical Perspective*, Harper Torchbooks, New York.

Cobb, M. 1998, 'Assessing spiritual need: An examination of practice', in M. Cobb & V. Robshaw (eds), *The Spiritual Challenge of Health Care*, Churchill Livingstone, Edinburgh, pp. 105–18.

—— 2001, *The Dying Soul: Spiritual Care at the End of Life*, Open University Press, Buckingham.

Costain Schou, K. & Hewison, J. 1999, *Experiencing Cancer: Quality of Life in Treatment*, Open University Press, Buckingham.

Delumeau, J. 1990, *Sin and Fear: The Emergence of a Western Guilt Culture 13th–18th Centuries*, St Martin's Press, New York.

Drewery, W., with McKenzie, W. 1999, 'Therapy and faith', in I. Parker (ed.), *Deconstructing Psychotherapy*, Sage, London, pp. 132–49.

Field, D. 1996, 'Awareness and modern dying', *Mortality*, vol. 1, pp. 255–65.

Fischer, C. 1985, *Individualizing Psychological Assessment*, Brooks/Cole Publishing, Monterey, California.

Foucault, M. 1973, *The Birth of the Clinic*, Tavistock, London.

Frank, A. 1995, *The Wounded Storyteller: Body, Illness, and Ethics*, University of Chicago Press, Chicago.

Hockley, J. 1997, 'The evolution of the hospice approach', in D. Clark, J. Hockley, & S. Ahmedzai (eds), *New Themes in Palliative Care*, Open University Press, Buckingham, pp. 84–100.

Irion, P. 1988, *Hospice and Ministry*, Abingdon, Nashville.

Irwin, H. 2000, 'The end: A view from parapsychology', in A. Kellehear (ed.), *Death and Dying in Australia*, Oxford University Press, Melbourne, pp. 342–54.

Jalland, P. 1997, *Death in the Victorian Family*, Oxford University Press, Oxford.

Kagawa-Singer, M. 1993, 'Redefining health: Living with cancer', *Social Science and Medicine*, vol. 37, no. 3, pp. 295–304.

Kastenbaum, R. 1975, 'Towards standards of care for the terminally ill: Part III—What standards exist today?' *Omega*, vol. 6, pp. 289–90.

Kellehear, A. 1999, *Health Promoting Palliative Care*, Oxford University Press, Melbourne.

—— 2000, 'Spirituality and palliative care: A model of needs', *Palliative Medicine*, vol. 14, pp. 149–55.

Klass, D. 1999, *The Spiritual Lives of Bereaved Parents*, Brunner/Mazel, Philadelphia.

Kolakowski, L. 1982, *Religion: If There is No God ... On God, the Devil, Sin and Other Worries of the So-called Philosophy of Religion*, Fontana, London.

Law, W. 1728, 1965, *A Serious Call to a Devout and Holy Life*, Fontana, London.

Maslow, A. 1964, *Religions, Values and Peak Experiences*, Ohio State University Press, Columbus.

Montgomery, C. 1991, 'The care-giving relationship: Paradoxical and transcendent aspects', *Journal of Transpersonal Psychology*, vol. 23, no. 2, pp. 91–104.

Palliative Care Australia 1999, *Standards for Palliative Care Provision* (3rd edn), <www.pallcare.org.au>.

Rumbold, B. 1986, *Helplessness and Hope: Pastoral Care in Terminal Illness*, SCM Press, London.

—— 1998, 'Implications of mainstreaming hospice into palliative care services', in J. Parker & S. Aranda (eds), *Palliative Care: Explorations and Challenges*, MacLennan & Petty, Sydney, pp. 3–20.

Saunders, C., Summers, D., and Teller, N. (eds) 1981, *Hospice: The Living Idea*, Edward Arnold, London.

Walter, T. 1994, *The Revival of Death*, Routledge, London.

—— 1997, 'The ideology and organisation of spiritual care: Three approaches', *Palliative Medicine*, vol. 11, pp. 21–30.

Weenolsen, P. 1996, *The Art of Dying*, St Martin's Press, New York.

Wilson, M. 1976, *Health is for People*, Darton, Longman & Todd, London.

Part 4

Guidelines for Spiritual Care

Summary

GUIDELINES CONCERNING SPIRITUALITY AND SPIRITUAL CARE IN PALLIATIVE CARE

This concluding part attempts to gather together some of the insights and themes that have emerged through the discussions of the previous chapters. It begins by reviewing the range of approaches to spiritual care that are being taken today, then suggests some guidelines that might affect the way such care is understood and offered.

The introduction to part 1 identified four broad strands or approaches to spiritual care in the health literature. Each of these strands has its own particular understanding of spiritual need and spiritual care.

- In the first strand spirituality is primarily about questions of identity—who am I when my sense of self is threatened or dissolved?—such that spiritual need is manifested as existential insecurity: anxiety, fear, guilt, or dread. These immediate spiritual needs are met by providing a supportive relationship until security can—hopefully—be restored.
- In the second strand spirituality is primarily about meaning. The meaning that formerly sustained a sense of purpose in life has been disrupted by changed circumstances; new meaning must be found. It is assumed that this will emerge through reflection on past experiences as people revise their life stories. Spiritual need is shown in a person's loss of meaning and purpose in life, a loss of vocation. Spiritual care is provided through skilled listening and support as people review their lives and fashion fresh meaning.
- The third strand sees spirituality in terms of people's alliances with particular frameworks of religious belief and communities of practice. Here

spiritual need appears as uncertainty about belonging to the religious community, often arising from uncertainty about beliefs, particularly those concerned with destiny and purpose. Spiritual need presents as loss of community and loss of hope. Spiritual care encourages people to maintain, revive or initiate connections with an appropriate religious community.

- The fourth strand is similar to the third, but rather than encouraging affiliation with religious communities it offers alternative spiritual belief systems and practices as a source of hope.

Clearly, these strands complement each other and are woven together in many approaches to spiritual care. Questions of identity may be addressed through life review or religious allegiance, for example. But identifying the strands in this way also illustrates how a healthcare context may shape its interest in spirituality.

- The first strand is found most often in contexts concerned about assessment: anxiety, fear, guilt, and dread are more easily identified than loss of vocation, loss of hope, loss of community. This strand is, however, less clear about how to respond to the existential needs that are identified, with the risk that the indicators of spiritual need may then be treated as emotions to be eased, so that spiritual care becomes very much like supportive counselling.

- The second strand, which sees spirituality as a quest for meaning, is better suited to contexts in which relationships can be built over a period of time. It is not surprising, for example, that life review is a spiritual care strategy most often associated with residential aged care. This approach, however, can place the responsibility for creating meaning squarely on the individual, who is expected to find meaning in memory and so retain a sense of self. However, this inner work may not be enough. We need to express and confirm our sense of self in the everyday world—a sense of self cannot exist solely as a construct of our memories. Some residential contexts that encourage life review paradoxically fail to create communities that permit expression of the selves that are identified through review.

- The third strand, which equates spirituality with religious belief, is best suited to contexts that maintain a clear distinction between the public duties of healthcare and private personal concerns. The former involves attention to the body while the latter, if a patient so chooses, may involve a practitioner from the appropriate religious community. Here, spiritual care by healthcare practitioners is undertaken principally by offering referrals to chaplains or other religious workers.

- The fourth strand, in which individuals are encouraged to undertake their own spiritual search, operates more informally. Individual healthcare practitioners, family members, or friends may suggest reading materials or recommend contacting a particular independent, often self-accredited, spiritual care practitioner.

The third strand that separates healthcare from religious interests was, until recently of course, the socially endorsed approach. Now, however, many of the new spiritualities have no hesitation in entering not only the territory formerly occupied by organised religion but also the territory of healthcare. Somatic spiritualities, spiritual healing methods, mind/body approaches, all blur previous conceptual boundaries and challenge Western understanding of science and religion. Clearly, the purpose of these new spiritualities is to name aspects of human experience that have been marginalised or neglected by modern healthcare, as well as by modern religion. This revisionist thrust of the contemporary spirituality literature is insufficiently recognised in most healthcare writings. It is evident that at least part of the value of talk about spirituality is precisely the fact that it has not (yet) been captured by clinical or religious interests.

DEFINING SPIRITUALITY

The health literature is, more than most, committed to definitions of spirituality, some complementary, some competing, all usually attempting to impose clarity as a first step in devising schemes for assessing spiritual need. Inevitably, these definitions reflect the interests and concerns of those who construct them rather than those whose experiences are being categorised. While the generality of current discussions of spirituality may be a frustration to some, the apparent clarity produced by definition can be misleading. Definitions privilege particular perspectives and particular ways of knowing. Many institutionally based approaches to spirituality, for example, are interested in obtaining assessments that rely upon observation and interview. Such assessments tend to concentrate on formal religious affiliations and indications of emotional adjustment to the situation, with little or no attention paid to the social and personal meaning of those affiliations or the diverse sources of emotional disturbance. (After all, having spiritual status assessed by a stranger may be a primary cause of a person's upset or resistance.) There is considerable evidence that the path of definition and measurement, because of its clinical objectives, fails to take account of both traditional religious insights and new possibilities emerging from changing social conditions. The definitions may select from the complex ways in which spirituality is discussed, but they cannot impose order on the discussions.

TALKING ABOUT SPIRITUALITY

Of course, what we see in healthcare discussions of spirituality reflects a renewed social awareness of spirituality in popular thought, business, education, and religion itself. Most discussions of spirituality use an uneasy selection of traditional religious terms or, equally uneasily, try to avoid traditional religious vocabularies altogether. Clearly, talking about spirituality puts us in something of a bind. If we use religious terms we find ourselves connected more closely than we might wish to the traditions that developed those terms. But if we try to avoid religious language altogether we struggle, finding ourselves extending or subverting the meanings of everyday words in an attempt to convey our insights and experience. This book exemplifies this dilemma. As Pam McGrath says (chapter 12), we need a new language.

GUIDELINES

With this introduction, and with the resources of this collection behind us, we put forward the following series of guidelines concerning spirituality and the practice of spiritual care in palliative care. Most are summarised from the preceding chapters, while some are developed from the insights and principles contained therein.

Spiritual needs and possibilities

- Spirituality names that which gives coherence and direction to a person's life and provides that person with a place in the world. Spirituality is usually expressed through relationships with particular locations and objects, with particular practices and beliefs, with oneself, with others, with communities, with the ecosystem, with transcendence (Lartey 1997, p. 113). Such a sense of connectedness is a recurring theme of this book, but is illustrated particularly in chapters 6 and 10. It can be seen as having both continuity (chapter 1) and discontinuity (chapters 3 and 12) with religious belief.

- Spiritual needs and possibilities can be located through the connections and lack of connections occurring in these everyday relationships. When significant connections that hold us in place in the world are threatened or disrupted, so is our spiritual integrity. Spiritual needs and possibilities therefore cannot be separated from other aspects of life.
- It is possible to map these connections and estrangements in another's web of relationships, but such an assessment should be the beginning of a conversation. Only the person in relationship can truly determine where their own needs and possibilities lie. That is, it may be possible to make an objective assessment of the resources available to another, but not to assess that person's spirituality. While a range of assessment tools is available (Center to Improve Care of the Dying 2001; Cobb 1998, 2001; Hall 1997), the danger in using such tools is that they will then mediate the relationship between person and carer. It is the relationship, not the assessment task, that should be primary.
- Spiritual care requires that people be approached as whole people and respected as the authority for their own spiritual lives.

Relationships in spiritual care

- Relationships that are not mutual, that is, not open to meeting another as another, cannot offer spiritual care. What such relationships represent as spiritual assessment remains at a psychological level, and the process of evaluation may even further compromise the subject's spiritual health (Walter 1997).
- Put positively, spiritual care occurs in mutual human relationships (chapters 3 and 8) that offer companionship (chapters 6, 7, and 8) through which everyday relationships and events can become the vehicles of spiritual meaning (chapter 12). A companion's expertise can be important (chapter 6), but unless offered in companionship that expertise may be unwelcome and of little use.
- Companionship involves accompanying another on a quest, which in turn requires that the companion have a questing attitude to life—be receptive to others' insights and open to possibility (chapter 13). Such a person-centred role, with its accompanying vulnerability and uncertainty, is not readily adopted by professional care-givers (Rumbold 1986; Hall 1997), and implies a need for ongoing formation.
- In spiritual care there are no expert solutions to be delivered, but well-developed expertise is needed in offering mutual relationship, attending

to the process of spiritual awareness, and assisting expression of spiritual insight (chapters 7 and 13). Pastoral care is one discipline that has sought to develop these skills, principally through the method of reflective practice. This is not an argument for pastoral care workers being the sole expert practitioners of spiritual care, but, rather, an argument for all palliative care disciplines to develop reflective practice.

Strategies for spiritual care

- Spiritual issues arise from situations and contexts that distract us or deprive us of what we need, personal narratives that no longer make sense of our present experience, and spiritualities incompatible with our own. Helpful responses include the following:
  - Minimising disruption to people's lives by paying attention to their continuing social identity and vocation rather than the patient role necessitated by illness, treatment, and care (Costain Schou & Hewison 1999). Spiritual care should resist the patient role, or at least work to keep it in proper perspective.
  - Supporting existing connections and encouraging new or neglected possibilities (discuss, for example, some of the roads not taken in that person's life).
  - Assessing the context (home and family, network of friends, institution) in which the person is attempting to maintain or develop spiritual awareness. Does the spirituality of this context support or resist this awareness? For example, is the person attempting to develop a quest spirituality in a context that is committed to restitution? Is their experience of chaos being diagnosed as a problem to be solved rather than a mystery to be entered? (chapters 5 and 13, Frank 1995).
  - Interventions in spiritual care in general involve addressing the person's situation, their story, or the systems of belief in which they participate (these are the three domains identified by Kellehear 2000).
- Because forming a mutual relationship is basic to spiritual care:
  - consider referral when such a relationship can't be formed
  - be sparing with referral when such a relationship already exists
  - be clear about the purposes of referral; for example, to refer a person to a religious practitioner does not obviate the need to continue offering spiritual care in other complementary ways.

- Because reflective practice is vital (Schön 1987),
  - undertake research (chapter 12)
  - practise journalling
  - seek peer supervision
  - arrange professional supervision
  - undertake formation in selected spiritual practices or a particular spiritual tradition.

Spiritual care in palliative care

- Maintaining a spiritual discourse is essential to maintaining the integrity of palliative care as a person-centred discipline. Spiritual care is perhaps the only domain of care where the patient's expertise and authority are recognised. (In the other domains, while patients are consulted, the options offered come from the expertise of others and outcomes are evaluated on external expert criteria.) Thus we need to reject attempts to capture spirituality in a professional discourse (through objective assessment, imposed terminology, etc.), while supporting and facilitating patients' own spiritual awareness and the actions and language that express this awareness.
- Research is an important tool for developing spiritual care (chapter 12, McGrath 1999). Not the least of the benefits of research is that it encourages us to pay systematic attention to our own context and practice, that is, to practise reflectively.

A public health approach is required (chapter 11), that is, everyone is responsible for spiritual care because it is a human, not merely a professional, responsibility. Spiritual care begins not in the final days of life, but in the communities in which we live and are formed as people. Part of the spiritual care task of palliative care is to tell the stories of people finding life in facing death in ways that society at large may hear.

REFERENCES

Center to Improve Care of the Dying 2001, <http://www.gwu.edu/~cicd/toolkit/spiritual.html>, 16 May.

Cobb, M. 1998, 'Assessing spiritual needs: An examination of practice', in M. Cobb & V. Robshaw (eds), *The Spiritual Challenge of Health Care*, Churchill Livingstone, Edinburgh, pp. 105–18.

—— 2001, *The Dying Soul: Spiritual Care at the End of Life*, Open University Press, Buckingham.

Costain Schou, K. & Hewison, J. 1999, *Experiencing Cancer: Quality of Life in Treatment*, Open University Press, Buckingham.

Frank, A. 1995, *The Wounded Storyteller: Body, Illness and Ethics*, Houghton Mifflin, Boston.

Hall, B. 1997, 'Spirituality in terminal illness: An alternative view of theory', *Journal of Holistic Nursing*, vol. 15, no. 1, pp. 82–96.

Kellehear, A. 2000, 'Spirituality and palliative care: A model of needs', *Palliative Medicine*, vol. 14, pp. 149–55.

Lartey, E. 1997, *In Living Colour: An Intercultural Approach to Pastoral Care and Counselling*, Cassell, London.

McGrath, P. 1999, 'Exploring spirituality through research: An important but challenging task', *Progress in Palliative Care*, vol. 7, no. 1, pp. 3–9.

Rumbold, B. 1986, *Helplessness and Hope: Pastoral Care in Terminal Illness*, SCM Press, London.

Schön, D. 1987, *Educating the Reflective Practitioner*, Jossey-Bass, San Francisco.

Walter, T. 1997, 'The ideology and organization of spiritual care: Three approaches', *Palliative Medicine*, vol. 11, no. 1, pp. 21–30.

Index